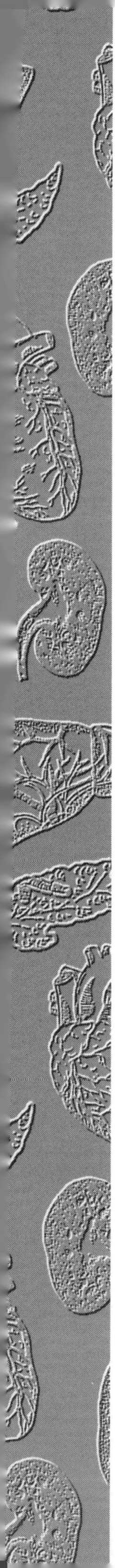



# Transplantation Drug Pocket Reference Guide

Second Edition

# Transplantation Drug Pocket Reference Guide

**Second Edition**

**Hans Sollinger, MD, PhD**
Folkert O. Belzer Professor of Surgery
Chairman, Division of Organ Transplantation
University of Wisconsin
Madison, Wisconsin, USA

**John Pirsch, MD**
Associate Professor of Medicine and Surgery
Director of Medical Transplantation
University of Wisconsin
Madison, Wisconsin, USA

LANDES
Bioscience Publishers

TRANSPLANTATION DRUG POCKET REFERENCE GUIDE

R.G. LANDES BIOSCIENCE PUBLISHERS
Austin, Texas, U.S.A.



Please address all inquiries to the Publishers:
R.G. Landes Company, 810 South Church Street, Georgetown, Texas, U.S.A. 78626
Phone: 512/ 863 7762; FAX: 512/ 863 0081

International and U.S. ISBN 1-57059-162-8

Although this pocket reference guide summarizes pertinent drug information, full Prescribing Information should be consulted before prescribing any product. The contents of this publication are the sole responsibility of the medical editors and not of Hoffman-La Roche or the Publisher.

While the authors, editors, and publisher believe that drug selection and dosage and the specifications and usage of equipment and devices, as set forth in this book, are in accord with current recommendations and practice at the time of publication, they make no warranty, expressed or implied, with respect to material described in this book. In view of the ongoing research, equipment development, changes in governmental regulations and the rapid accumulation of information relating to the biomedical sciences, the reader is urged to carefully review and evaluate the information provided herein.

**Library of Congress Cataloging-in-Publication Data**

Transplantation drug pocket reference guide [edited by] Hans Sollinger, Jonathan Pirsch. Second Edition

p. cm. ISBN 1-57059-162-8 (soft cover)

1. Transplantation of organs, tissues, etc.—Complications—Chemotherapy—Handbooks, manuals, etc. I. Sollinger, Hans.

[DNLM: 1. Drug Therapy—handbooks. 2. Transplantation—handbooks. 3. Immunosuppressive Agents—pharmacology—handbooks. 4. Anti-Infective Agents—pharmacology—handbooks. 5. Postoperative Complications—drug therapy—handbooks. WB 39 T772 1994]

RM301.T73 1994
615.5'8—dc20
DNLM/DLC 94-7784
for Library of Congress CIP

# Table of Contents

# Introduction

The field of transplantation continues to evolve. In the years since the first publication of the ***Transplantation Drug Pocket Reference Guide***, the therapeutic armamentarium for transplantation has grown. The introduction of new agents continues to enhance our ability to improve the short- and long-term success of transplantation.

The second edition of the ***Transplantation Drug Pocket Reference Guide*** includes information on agents recently approved for use in transplant recipients. As in the first edition, we compiled practical information on the wide array of pharmaceutical agents currently available—both those used for immunosuppression and those used to minimize posttransplant complications. The agents described here are the most frequently prescribed drugs in the Transplant Service at the University of Wisconsin. We hope you find this information to be useful and practical in managing the transplant patient.

# Chapter 1

# Working Guide to Immunosuppression

## Current Agents Overview

- Antithymocyte Globulin
- Azathioprine
- Cyclophosphamide
- Cyclosporine-A
- Cyclosporine Capsules and Oral Solution for Microemulsion
- Methylprednisolone
- Muromonab-CD3
- Mycophenolate Mofetil
- Prednisone
- Tacrolimus (FK-506)

## Investigational Agents

- Rapamycin (sirolimus)
- 15-Deoxyspergualin

# Current Agents Overview

| Agent | Dosage |
|---|---|
| **Antithymocyte Globulin** | *Delaying Onset of Allograft Rejection*<br>• Fixed dose of 15 mg/kg/d IV for 7 to 14 days<br>• First dose should be administered within 24 hours before or after transplantation<br><br>*Treatment of Rejection*<br>• 10 mg/kg/d IV to 15 mg/kg/d IV for 14 days |
| **Azathioprine** | • 3 mg/kg/d to 5 mg/kg/d single dose given at time of transplantation<br>• 1 mg/kg/d to 3 mg/kg/d for maintenance<br>• Dose usually adjusted depending on WBCs<br>• Lower doses should be considered in presence of renal dysfunction |
| **Cyclophosphamide** | • 2 mg/kg/d to 3 mg/kg/d is initial recommended dose, but is rapidly reduced due to toxicity |
| **Cyclosporine-A** | *Gelatin Capsules & Oral Solution*<br>• 15 mg/kg single dose given 4 to 12 hours prior to transplantation<br>• Single daily dose is continued postoperatively for 1 to 2 weeks and then tapered by 5% each week until maintenance dose of 5 mg/kg/d to 10 mg/kg/d is reached<br><br>*IV Infusion*<br>• 5 mg/kg to 6 mg/kg single dose given 4 to 12 hours prior to transplantation<br>• Single daily IV dose continued postoperatively until patient can tolerate oral formulations |
| **Cyclosporine Capsules and Oral Solution for Microemulsion** | **NOTE: Neoral and Sandimmune are not bioequivalent and should not be used interchangeably. Neoral has increased bioavailability and this should be taken into consideration when making dosing decisions.**<br><br>• Daily dose should be given as two divided doses on a consistent schedule<br><br>*Newly Transplanted Patients*<br>• Initial dose of Neoral should be the same as a Sandimmune dose. Suggested initial doses include:<br>– 9 ± 3 mg/kg/day for kidney transplant patients<br>– 8 ± 4 mg/kg/day for liver transplant patients<br>– 7 ± 3 mg/kg/day for heart transplant patients<br>• The dose is then subsequently adjusted to achieve a predefined cyclosporine blood concentration<br><br>*Conversion from Sandimmune to Neoral*<br>• Neoral should be started with the same daily dose as was previously used with Sandimmune (1:1 dose conversion)<br>• The Neoral dose should then be adjusted to achieve preconversion cyclosporine blood trough concentrations<br>• Until cyclosporine blood trough concentrations reach preconversion levels, monitoring should be undertaken every 4 to 7 days |

*Continued ...*

# Current Agents Overview

| Agent | Dosage |
|---|---|
| **Methylprednisolone** | *Induction*<br>• 250 mg to 1000 mg at time of transplantation and for next 2 to 3 doses<br><br>*Taper*<br>• Start at 2 mg/kg/d, taper to a range of 0.15 mg/kg/d to 0.2 mg/kg/d after one year<br><br>*Attenuation of Cytokine Release Syndrome*<br>• 8 mg/kg given 1 to 4 hours prior to first injection of muromonab-CD3 |
| **Muromonab-CD3** | • 5 mg/d IV for 10 to 14 days |
| **Mycophenolate Mofetil** | Initial dose should be given within 72 hours following transplantation<br>• 1.0 g twice a day used in combination with corticosteroids and cyclosporine |
| **Prednisone** | *Maintenance—Adults*<br>• 0.1 mg/kg/d to 2 mg/kg/d usually given once daily<br><br>*Maintenance—Pediatric*<br>• 0.25 mg/kg/d to 2 mg/kg/d or 25 mg/m$^2$ to 60 mg/m$^2$ usually given daily or on alternate days |
| **Tacrolimus (FK-506)** | *IV Infusion*<br>• 0.05 mg/kg/d to 0.10 mg/kg/d administered no sooner than 6 hours posttransplantation<br><br>*Capsules*<br>• 0.15 mg/kg/d to 0.30 mg/kg/d administered in 2 divided daily doses every 12 hours<br>• First dose should be given 8 to 12 hours after discontinuing IV infusion |

# Antithymocyte Globulin (Equine)

| | |
|---|---|
| **Brand Name** | ATGAM® |
| **Company** | Pharmacia & Upjohn, Inc. |
| **Class** | • Immunosuppressant gamma globulin, primarily monomeric IgG, from hyperimmune serum of horses immunized with human thymic lymphocytes |
| **Mechanism of Action** | • Antibodies of multiple specificities interact with lymphocyte surface antigens, depleting numbers of circulating, thymus-dependent lymphocytes and interfering with cell-mediated and humoral immune responses |
| **Indications** | • Management of renal allograft rejection<br>• Adjunct to other immunosuppressive therapy to delay the onset of the first rejection episode |
| **Contraindication** | • Hypersensitivity to ATGAM or any other equine gamma globulin preparation |
| **Warnings** | • Should be administered in facilities equipped and staffed with adequate laboratory and supportive medical resources<br>• Immunosuppressive activity may vary from lot to lot<br>• Potential for the transmission of infectious agents<br>• Treatment should be discontinued if the following occur:<br>• Symptoms of anaphylaxis • Thrombocytopenia • Leukopenia |
| **Special Precautions** | • Risk of infection, leukopenia, and thrombocytopenia<br>• Safety and effectiveness demonstrated only in patients who received concomitant immunosuppression<br>• Pregnancy Category C |
| **Adverse Reactions** | • Fever (1 patient in 3)<br>• Chills (1 patient in 7)<br>• Leukopenia (1 patient in 7)<br>• Dermatologic reactions (1 patient in 8)<br>• Thrombocytopenia (1 patient in 9)<br><br>*Reported in >1%, but <5% of Patients*<br>• Arthralgia<br>• Clotted A/V fistula<br>• Night sweats<br>• Peripheral thrombophlebitis<br>• Chest and/or back pain<br>• Nausea and/or vomiting<br>• Pain at infusion site<br>• Stomatitis |
| **Drug Interaction** | • Dextrose Injection, USP |
| **Formulation** | • 5 mL ampule containing 50 mg/mL |
| **Dosage** | *Delaying Onset of Allograft Rejection*<br>• Fixed dose of 15 mg/kg/d IV for 7 to 14 days<br>• First dose should be administered within 24 hours before or after transplantation<br><br>*Treatment of Rejection*<br>• 10 mg/kg/d IV to 15 mg/kg/d IV for 14 days<br>A dose should not be infused in less than 4 hours |

*Editors' Notes:*

There are several antilymphocyte preparations used worldwide. In addition to ATGAM (Pharmacia & Upjohn), horse MALG (University of Minnesota) and rabbit Fresenius ATG (Fresenius Company, Germany) are used. Fresenius ATG is not FDA approved, but clinical trials are in progress. MALG is not currently available and its future status is questionable. All ALG preparations seem to have similar efficacy and side effects. ATGAM and MALG are administered via a central line. Fresenius ATG can be given via peripheral IV. The major side effects include skin eruptions and bone marrow suppression. The use of antilymphocyte therapy may also lead to a higher incidence of CMV and EBV infection.

# Azathioprine

| | |
|---|---|
| **Brand Name** | Imuran® |
| **Company** | Glaxo Wellcome Inc. |
| **Class** | • Immunosuppressive antimetabolite (6-mercaptopurine) |
| **Mechanism of Action** | • Interferes with DNA and RNA synthesis, thereby inhibiting differentiation and proliferation of both T and B lymphocytes |
| **Indication** | • Adjunct for the prevention of rejection in renal homotransplantation |
| **Clinical Experience** | • 35% to 55% 5-year patient survival in over 16,000 transplantations |
| **Contraindication** | • Hypersensitivity to azathioprine |
| **Warnings** | • Increased risk of neoplasia<br>• Severe myelosuppression<br>• Serious infection<br>• Pregnancy Category D |
| **Special Precautions** | • Gastrointestinal hypersensitivity reaction<br>• Periodic blood counts may be needed |
| **Adverse Reactions** | • Leukopenia (>50%)<br>• Infection (20%)<br>• Nausea and vomiting (NA)<br>• Neoplasia (3.3%)<br>• Hepatotoxicity (NA) |
| **Drug Interactions** | • **Allopurinol**<br>• Agents affecting myelopoiesis<br>• Angiotensin converting enzyme inhibitors |
| **Formulations** | • 50 mg scored tablets<br>• 20 mL vial containing 100 mg azathioprine |
| **Dosage** | • 3 mg/kg/d to 5 mg/kg/d single dose given at time of transplantation<br>• 1 mg/kg/d to 3 mg/kg/d for maintenance<br>• Dose usually adjusted depending on WBCs<br>• Lower doses should be considered in presence of renal dysfunction |

***Editors' Notes:***

Combined administration of azathioprine and allopurinol may result in severe pancytopenia. Azathioprine may cause liver dysfunction, frequently manifested by an isolated rise in ALT and bilirubin. With the introduction of mycophenolate mofetil, azathioprine may be relegated to a second-line antimetabolite for the prevention of graft rejection.

# Cyclophosphamide

| | |
|---|---|
| **Brand Name** | Cytoxan® |
| **Company** | Bristol-Myers Oncology Division |
| **Class** | • Immunosuppressive antimetabolite |
| **Mechanism of Action** | • Interferes with the growth of susceptible, rapidly proliferating cells, possibly through cross-linking of cellular DNA |
| **Application in Transplantation** | • Adjunct to other immunosuppressive therapy to delay onset of first rejection episode |
| **Contraindications** | • Severe myelosuppression<br>• Hypersensitivity to cyclophosphamide |
| **Warnings** | • Risk of myeloproliferative and lymphoproliferative malignancies<br>• Fetal damage • Sterility in both sexes<br>• Amenorrhea • Oligospermia or azoospermia<br>• Hemorrhagic cystitis • Urinary bladder fibrosis<br>• Cardiotoxicity at high doses (120 mg/kg to 270 mg/kg)<br>• Risk of infection |
| **Special Precautions** | • Treatment should be discontinued if any of the following are present:<br>• leukopenia<br>• thrombocytopenia<br>• previous exposure to other cytotoxic agents<br>• impaired renal function<br>• impaired hepatic function<br>• Hematologic profile and urine should be monitored periodically<br>• Should be used with caution in adrenalectomized patients<br>• Pregnancy Category D |
| **Adverse Reactions** | • Sterility in both sexes • Oligospermia or azoospermia<br>• Nausea and vomiting • Leukopenia<br>• Alopecia • Hemorrhagic cystitis<br>• Urinary bladder fibrosis • Renal tubular necrosis<br>• Opportunistic infection |
| **Drug Interactions** | • Phenobarbitol<br>• Succinylcholine<br>• Anesthesiologist should be informed if patient is to receive general anesthesia within 10 days of treatment |
| **Formulations** | *Cytoxan for Injection*<br>• 100 mg vial<br>• 200 mg vial<br>• 500 mg vial<br>• 1.0 g vial<br>• 2.0 g vial<br><br>*Lyophilized Cytoxan for Injection*<br>• 100 mg vial<br>• 200 mg vial<br>• 500 mg vial<br>• 1.0 g vial<br>• 2.0 g vial |
| **Dosage** | • 2 mg/kg/d to 3 mg/kg/d is initial recommended dose, but is rapidly reduced due to toxicity |

*Editors' Notes:*

Cyclophosphamide is given in patients with contraindications to azathioprine. The dose is usually half of the azathioprine dose. Prolonged use of cyclophosphamide is not recommended due to the possibility of future malignancy.

Immuno-suppression | Antimicrobials | Cardiovascular Agents | Antiosteo-porosis Agents | Antiplatelets | Diabetes Agents | Ulcer Treatment | Diuretics | Other Agents

# Cyclosporine-A

| | |
|---|---|
| **Brand Name** | Sandimmune® |
| **Company** | Novartis |
| **Class** | • Immunosuppressant produced as a metabolite by the fungus species *Tolypocladium inflatum* Gams |
| **Mechanism of Action** | • Preferential inhibition of T lymphocytes<br>• Suppresses activation of T lymphocytes by inhibiting production and release of lymphokines, specifically interleukin-2 |
| **Indications** | • Prophylaxis of graft rejection in kidney, liver, and heart allogeneic transplantation<br>• Treatment of chronic rejection previously treated with other immuno-suppressants |
| **Contraindication** | • Hypersensitivity to cyclosporine or polyoxyethylated castor oil |
| **Warnings** | • Nephrotoxicity<br>• Hepatotoxicity<br>• Increased susceptibility to infection and lymphoma<br>• Erratic absorption of soft gelatin capsules and oral solution necessitates repeated monitoring of cyclosporine blood levels<br>• Anaphylactic reactions with IV formulation |
| **Special Precautions** | • Hypertension may occur and require therapy with antihypertensives (potassium-sparing diuretics should not be used)<br>• Repeated laboratory monitoring is required<br>• Pregnancy Category C |
| **Adverse Reactions** | • Renal dysfunction (25% - renal, 38% - cardiac, 37% - hepatic)<br>• Tremor (21% - renal, 31% - cardiac, 55% - hepatic)<br>• Hirsutism (21% - renal, 28% - cardiac, 45% - hepatic)<br>• Hypertension (13% - renal, 53% - cardiac, 27% - hepatic)<br>• Gum hyperplasia ( 9% - renal, 5% - cardiac, 16% - hepatic) |
| **Drug Interactions** | *Drugs with Synergistic Nephrotoxicity*<br>• Gentamicin • Amphotericin B • Tobramycin<br>• Ketoconazole • Vancomycin • Melphalan<br>• Cimetidine • TMP-SMX • Ranitidine<br>• Azapropazon • Diclofenac<br><br>*Drugs that Increase Cyclosporine Levels*<br>• Diltiazem • Ketoconazole • Nicardipine<br>• Erythromycin • Verapamil • Itraconazole<br>• Danazol • Bromocriptine • Fluconazole<br>• Methylprednisolone • Metoclopramide<br><br>*Drugs that Decrease Cyclosporine Levels*<br>• Rifampin • Phenobarbitol<br>• Carbamazepine • Phenytoin<br><br>*Reduced Clearance with Cyclosporine*<br>• Prednisone<br>• Lovastatin<br>• Digoxin<br><br>*Other*<br>• Vaccinations—live vaccinations should be avoided |

*Continued ...*

# Cyclosporine-A

| | |
|---|---|
| **Formulations** | • 25 mg soft gelatin capsules<br>• 50 mL bottle containing 100 mg/mL for oral solution<br>• 5 mL vial containing 50 mg/mL |
| **Dosage** | *Gelatin Capsules & Oral Solution*<br>• 15 mg/kg single dose given 4 to 12 hours prior to transplantation<br>• Single daily dose is continued postoperatively for 1 to 2 weeks and then tapered by 5% each week until maintenance dose of 5 mg/kg/d to 10 mg/kg/d is reached<br><br>*IV Infusion*<br>• 5 mg/kg to 6 mg/kg single dose given 4 to 12 hours prior to transplantation<br>• Single daily IV dose continued postoperatively until patient can tolerate oral formulations |

*Editors' Notes:*

Recent evidence suggests higher doses of cyclosporine-A and higher blood levels may prolong graft survival and improve renal function.

# Cyclosporine Capsules and Oral Solution for Microemulsion

| | |
|---|---|
| **Brand Name** | Neoral® |
| **Company** | Novartis |
| **Class** | • Immunosuppressant produced as a metabolite by the fungus species *Tolypocladium inflatum* Gams |
| **Mechanism of Action** | • Preferential inhibition of T lymphocytes<br>• Suppresses activation of T lymphocytes by inhibiting production and release of lymphokines, specifically interleukin-2 |
| **Indications** | • Prophylaxis of graft rejection in kidney, liver, and heart allogeneic transplantation |
| **Contraindication** | • Hypersensitivity to cyclosporine or any of the ingredients of the formulation |
| **Warnings** | • Nephrotoxicity<br>• Hepatotoxicity<br>• Increased susceptibility to infection and lymphoma<br>• Reports of nephrotoxicity in pediatric and adult patients, especially when used in conjunction with methylprednisolone<br>• Neoral is not bioequivalent to Sandimmune® |
| **Special Precautions** | • Any change in cyclosporine formulation should be made cautiously and under the advisement of a physician—Patients should be given detailed dosage instructions<br>• Hypertension may occur and require therapy with antihypertensives (potassium-sparing diuretics should not be used)<br>• Repeated laboratory monitoring is required<br>• Pregnancy Category C |
| **Adverse Reactions** | • Renal dysfunction<br>• Tremor<br>• Hirsutism<br>• Hypertension<br>• Gum hyperplasia |
| **Drug Interactions** | *Drugs With Synergistic Nephrotoxicity*<br>• Gentamicin • Amphotericin B<br>• Tobramycin • Ketoconazole<br>• Vancomycin • Melphalan<br>• TMP-SMX • Tacrolimus<br>• Cimetidine • Diclofenac<br>• Ranitidine • Azapropazon<br><br>*Drugs That Increase Cyclosporine Levels*<br>• Diltiazem • Clarithromycin<br>• Nicardipine • Allopurinol<br>• Verapamil • Danazol<br>• Ketoconazole • Bromocriptine<br>• Fluconazole • Methylprednisolone<br>• Itraconazole • Metoclopramide<br>• Erythromycin |

*Continued ...*

# Cyclosporine Capsules and Oral Solution for Microemulsion

| | |
|---|---|
| **Drug Interactions** (continued) | *Drugs that Decrease Cyclosporine Levels*<br>• Rifampin<br>• Nafcillin<br>• Phenytoin<br>• Phenobarbitol<br>• Carbamazepine<br>• Octreotide<br>• Ticlopidine<br><br>*Reduced Clearance with Cyclosporine*<br>• Prednisone<br>• Digoxin<br>• Lovastatin<br><br>*Other*<br>• Vaccinations—live vaccinations should be avoided |
| **Formulations** | • Soft gelatin capsules for microemulsion<br>• Oral solution for microemulsion |
| **Dosage** | **NOTE: Neoral and Sandimmune are not bioequivalent and should not be used interchangeably. Neoral has increased bioavailability and this should be taken into consideration when making dosing decisions.**<br><br>• Daily dose should be given as two divided doses on a consistent schedule<br><br>*Newly Transplanted Patients*<br>• Initial dose of Neoral should be the same as a Sandimmune dose. Suggested initial doses include:<br>– 9 ± 3 mg/kg/day for kidney transplant patients<br>– 8 ± 4 mg/kg/day for liver transplant patients<br>– 7 ± 3 mg/kg/day for heart transplant patients<br>• The dose is then subsequently adjusted to achieve a predefined cyclosporine blood concentration<br><br>*Conversion from Sandimmune to Neoral*<br>• Neoral should be started with the same daily dose as was previously used with Sandimmune (1:1 dose conversion)<br>• The Neoral dose should then be adjusted to achieve preconversion cyclosporine blood trough concentrations<br>• Until cyclosporine blood trough concentrations reach preconversion levels, monitoring should be undertaken every 4 to 7 days |

*Editors' Notes:*

Neoral is a new microemulsion formulation of cyclosporine-A. Advantages include a more predictable pharmacokinetic profile and better absorption patterns. Trough cyclosporine levels correlate more closely with total drug exposure, which may be clinically relevant.

# Methylprednisolone

| | |
|---|---|
| **Brand Name** | Solu-Medrol® |
| **Company** | Pharmacia and Upjohn, Inc. |
| **Class** | • Anti-inflammatory steroid |
| **Mechanism of Action** | • Causes emigration of circulating T cells from intravascular tissue compartment to lymphoid tissue<br>• Inhibits production of T-cell lymphokines that are needed to amplify macrophage and lymphocyte response |
| **Applications in Transplantation** | • Immunosuppressive adjunct for the prevention and treatment of solid organ rejection<br>• Attenuation of cytokine release syndrome in patients treated with muromonab-CD3 |
| **Contraindications** | • Hypersensitivity to methylprednisolone and/or its components<br>• Systemic fungal infections<br>• Prematurity in infants |
| **Warnings** | • May produce posterior subcapsular cataracts, glaucoma, and may enhance the establishment of secondary ocular infections due to fungi or viruses<br>• Increased calcium excretion<br>• Vaccination should not be undertaken during therapy<br>• Cardiac arrhythmias, circulatory collapse, and/or cardiac arrest have occurred after rapid administration<br>• Adequate human reproduction studies have not been undertaken |
| **Special Precautions** | • Use with caution in patients with hypothyroidism, cirrhosis, ocular herpes simplex, hypertension, congestive heart failure, and ulcerative colitis<br>• Psychologic derangements may occur while on therapy |
| **Adverse Reactions** | • Sodium and fluid retention, congestive heart failure in susceptible patients, potassium loss, hypokalemic alkalosis, hypertension<br>• Muscle weakness, steroid myopathy, loss of muscle mass, severe arthralgia, vertebral compression fractures, aseptic necrosis of humeral and femoral heads, pathologic fracture of long bones, osteoporosis<br>• Peptic ulcer with possible perforation and hemorrhage, pancreatitis, abdominal distension, ulcerative esophagitis<br>• Impaired wound healing, thin fragile skin, petechiae and ecchymoses, facial erythema, increased sweating, suppressed reaction to skin tests<br>• Pseudotumor cerebri, convulsions, vertigo, headache<br>• Cushingoid state, suppression of growth in children, secondary adrenocortical and pituitary unresponsiveness, menstrual irregularities, decreased carbohydrate tolerance, manifestations of latent diabetes mellitus, increased requirements for insulin or oral hypoglycemic agent<br>• Posterior subcapsular cataracts, increased intraocular pressure, glaucoma, exophthalmos |
| **Drug Interactions** | • Barbiturates • Phenytoin • Rifampin<br>• Salicylates • Vaccines • Toxoids |

*Continued ...*

# Methylprednisolone

| | |
|---|---|
| **Formulations** | • 40 mg single dose vial<br>• 125 mg single dose vial<br>• 500 mg vial<br>• 500 mg vial with diluent<br>• 1 g vial<br>• 1 g vial with diluent |
| **Dosage** | *Induction*<br>• 250 mg to 1000 mg at time of transplantation and for next 2 to 3 doses<br><br>*Taper*<br>• Start at 2 mg/kg/d, taper to a range of 0.15 mg/kg/d to 0.2 mg/kg/d after one year<br><br>*Attenuation of Cytokine Release Syndrome*<br>• 8 mg/kg given 1 to 4 hours prior to first injection of muromonab-CD3 |

*Editors' Notes:*

Multiple different regimens of methylprednisolone have been utilized to treat rejection. The initial higher doses are the most important in controlling rejection. It is unclear whether prolonged tapering of steroids following rejection is of value.

# Muromonab-CD3

| | |
|---|---|
| **Brand Name** | ORTHOCLONE OKT®3 |
| **Company** | Ortho Biotech Inc. |
| **Class** | • Immunosuppressive monoclonal antibody with singular specificity to CD3 antigen of human T cells |
| **Mechanism of Action** | • Blocks the function of CD3 molecule in the membrane of human T cells, which has been associated in vitro with the antigen recognition structure of human T cells that is essential for signal transduction |
| **Indications** | • Treatment of acute renal allograft rejection as soon as it is diagnosed<br>• Treatment of steroid-resistant acute cardiac allograft rejection<br>• Treatment of steroid-resistant acute hepatic allograft rejection |
| **Contraindications** | • Hypersensitivity to muromonab-CD3 and/or any product of murine origin<br>• Antimurine antibody titers ≥1:1000<br>• Uncompensated heart failure or fluid overload<br>• History of seizures<br>• Determined to be or suspected of being pregnant or breast-feeding |
| **Warnings** | • Cytokine release syndrome, ranging from a mild, self-limited, flu-like syndrome to a less-frequently reported severe, life-threatening shock-like reaction, has been associated with first few doses<br>  • Can be attenuated by premedicating with methylprednisolone, 8 mg/kg, given 1 to 4 hours prior to first injection<br>• Anaphylactic reactions<br>• Neuropsychiatric events, including seizures, encephalopathy, cerebral edema, aseptic meningitis, and headache<br>• Risk of infection and neoplasia<br>• Patients should be managed in a facility equipped and staffed for cardiopulmonary resuscitation |
| **Special Precautions** | • Clear chest X ray and weight restriction of ≤3% above patient's minimum weight during the week prior to injection<br>• If patient's temperature exceeds 37.8°C, it should be lowered with antipyretics before each injection<br>• Periodic monitoring to ensure muromonab-CD3 levels >800 ng/mL and $CD3^+$ cell levels <25 cell/$mm^3$<br>• Potentially serious signs and symptoms with immediate onset are likely due to hypersensitivity and therapy should be discontinued<br>• Antiseizure precautions should be undertaken<br>• Patient should be monitored for signs of infection and/or lymphoproliferative disorders<br>• Antimurine antibody titers should be monitored after therapy with muromonab-CD3<br>• As with other immunosuppressives, arterial or venous thromboses of allografts and other vascular beds have been reported<br>• Pregnancy Category C |

*Continued ...*

# Muromonab-CD3

| | |
|---|---|
| **Adverse Reactions** | • Pyrexia<br>• Chills<br>• Dyspnea<br>• Nausea and vomiting<br>• Chest pain<br>• Diarrhea<br>• Tremor<br>• Wheezing<br>• Headache<br>• Hypersensitivity reactions<br>• Tachycardia<br>• Rigor<br>• Hypertension<br>• Infection with herpes simplex virus, cytomegalovirus, *Staphylococcus epidermidis, Pneumocystis carinii, Legionella, Cryptococcus, Serratia,* and gram-negative bacteria<br>• Posttransplant lymphoproliferative disorders |
| **Drug Interactions** | • Indomethacin alone and in conjunction with muromonab-CD3 has been associated with CNS effects<br>• Corticosteroids alone and in conjunction with muromonab-CD3 have been associated with psychosis and infection<br>• Azathioprine alone and in conjunction with muromonab-CD3 has been associated with infection and malignancies<br>• Cyclosporine-A alone and in conjunction with muromonab-CD3 has been associated with seizures, encephalopathy, infection, malignancies, and thrombotic events |
| **Formulation** | • 5 mL ampule containing 5 mg |
| **Dosage** | • 5 mg/d IV for 10 to 14 days |

*Editors' Notes:*

Recent evidence suggests that giving 250 mg of methylprednisolone 6 hours prior and 1 hour prior to administration of muromonab-CD3 can decrease the incidence of cytokine release syndrome (CRS). Pentoxifylline has not been shown to attenuate CRS. Indomethacin, however, can be effective.

If CD3 levels remain high during therapy with muromonab-CD3, the dose may be increased or one may switch to an alternate antilymphocyte preparation.

Adjunctive prophylaxis with ganciclovir in CMV-positive patients or in recipients of CMV-positive organs may be effective in reducing risk of CMV infection.

# Mycophenolate Mofetil

| | |
|---|---|
| **Brand Name** | CellCept® |
| **Company** | Roche Laboratories |
| **Class** | • Immunosuppressive antimetabolite |
| **Mechanism of Action** | • Selectively inhibits inosine monophosphate dehydrogenase in the denovo pathway of purine synthesis, producing potent cytostatic effects on T and B lymphocytes |
| **Indication** | • Prophylaxis of graft rejection in patients receiving renal allogeneic transplantation |
| **Contraindication** | • Hypersensitivity to mycophenolate mofetil, mycophenolic acid or any components of the drug |
| **Warnings** | • Increased susceptibility to infection and lymphoma<br>• Adverse effects on fetal development have been observed in pregnant rats and rabbits—mycophenolate mofetil should not be used in pregnant women and contraception should be used during therapy<br>• Neutropenia has been observed |
| **Special Precaution** | • Gastrointestinal hemorrhage may occur<br>• Patients with renal impairment have shown higher MPA and MPAG AUCs than normal volunteers<br>• Should not be used in conjunction with azathioprine<br>• Repeated laboratory monitoring is required<br>• Pregnancy Category C |
| **Adverse Reactions** | • Diarrhea<br>• Leukopenia<br>• Sepsis<br>• Vomiting |
| **Drug Interactions** | • Acyclovir<br>• Antacids with magnesium and aluminum hydroxides<br>• Cholestyramine<br>• Drugs that alter gastrointestinal flora may interact with mycophenolate mofetil by disrupting enterohepatic recirculation<br>• Probenecid |
| **Formulation** | • 250-mg capsules supplied in bottles of 100 and 500 |
| **Dosage** | • 1.0 g twice a day used in combination with corticosteroids and cyclosporine<br>• Initial dose should be given within 72 hours following transplantation |

*Editors' Notes:*

Mycophenolate mofetil reduces the risk of first acute rejection by 50%. Toxicity is minor, but includes bone marrow suppression and gastrointestinal complaints. A higher incidence of CMV disease compared to azathioprine control was observed in the clinical trials.

# Prednisone

| | | | |
|---|---|---|---|
| **Brand Name** | Deltasone® | | |
| **Company** | Pharmacia and Upjohn, Inc. | | |
| **Class** | • Anti-inflammatory steroid | | |
| **Mechanism of Action** | • Causes emigration of circulating T cells from intravascular tissue compartment to lymphoid tissue<br>• Inhibits production of T cell lymphokines that are needed to amplify macrophage and lymphocyte response | | |
| **Application in Transplantation** | • Immunosuppressive adjunct for the prevention and treatment of solid organ rejection | | |
| **Contraindications** | • Hypersensitivity to prednisone and/or its components<br>• Systemic fungal infection | | |
| **Warnings** | • May produce posterior subcapsular cataracts, glaucoma, and may enhance the establishment of secondary ocular infections due to fungi or viruses<br>• Increased calcium excretion<br>• Vaccination should not be undertaken during therapy<br>• Adequate human reproduction studies have not been undertaken | | |
| **Special Precautions** | • Use with caution in patients with hypothyroidism, cirrhosis, ocular herpes simplex, hypertension, congestive heart failure, and ulcerative colitis<br>• Psychologic derangements may occur while on therapy | | |
| **Adverse Reactions** | • Sodium and fluid retention, congestive heart failure in susceptible patients, potassium loss, hypokalemic alkalosis, hypertension<br>• Muscle weakness, steroid myopathy, loss of muscle mass, vertebral compression fractures, aseptic necrosis of humeral and femoral heads, pathologic fracture of long bones, osteoporosis<br>• Peptic ulcer with possible perforation and hemorrhage, pancreatitis, abdominal distension, ulcerative esophagitis<br>• Impaired wound healing, thin fragile skin, petechiae and ecchymoses, facial erythema, increased sweating, suppressed reaction to skin tests<br>• Pseudotumor cerebri, convulsions, vertigo, headache<br>• Cushingoid state, suppression of growth in children, secondary adrenocortical and pituitary unresponsiveness, menstrual irregularities, decreased carbohydrate tolerance, manifestations of latent diabetes mellitus, increased requirements for insulin or oral hypoglycemic agent<br>• Posterior subcapsular cataracts, increased intraocular pressure, glaucoma, exophthalmos | | |
| **Drug Interactions** | • Barbiturates<br>• Salicylates | • Phenytoin<br>• Vaccines | • Rifampin<br>• Toxoids |
| **Dosage Strengths** | • 2.5 mg tablets<br>• 20 mg tablets | • 5 mg tablets<br>• 50 mg tablets | • 10 mg tablets |
| **Dosage** | *Maintenance—Adults*<br>• 0.1 mg/kg/d to 2 mg/kg/d usually given once daily<br><br>*Maintenance—Pediatric*<br>• 0.25 mg/kg/d to 2 mg/kg/d or 25 mg/m$^2$ to 60 mg/m$^2$ usually given daily or on alternate days | | |

*Editors' Notes:*

After rejection of a renal transplant, empirical weaning of prednisone over several weeks is recommended. If the patient develops fever, malaise, and graft tenderness, the transplanted kidney should be removed.

# Tacrolimus (FK-506)

| | |
|---|---|
| **Brand Name** | Prograf® |
| **Company** | Fujisawa |
| **Class** | • Macrolide antibiotic with immunosuppressant properties |
| **Mechanism of Action** | • Binds to a T-cell binding protein and prevents synthesis of interleukin-2 and other lymphokines essential to T-lymphocyte function |
| **Indications** | • Prophylaxis of graft rejection in liver allogeneic transplantation<br>• It is recommended that tacrolimus be used concomitantly with adrenal corticosteroids |
| **Contraindications** | • Hypersensitivity to tacrolimus<br>• Hypersensitivity to HCO-60 (polyoxyl 60 hydrogenated castor oil) |
| **Warnings** | • Neurotoxicity<br>• Nephrotoxicity<br>• Hyperkalemia<br>• Increased risk of infection and lymphomas<br>• Patients should be monitored closely for at least the first 30 minutes of therapy for signs of anaphylactic reactions |
| **Precautions** | • Hypertension is a common occurrence with tacrolimus and may require treatment with antihypertensive agents. Since tacrolimus may cause hyperkalemia, potassium-sparing diuretics should be avoided<br>• Hyperglycemia may occur and require treatment<br>• Lower doses should be used in patients with renal insufficiencies<br>• Patients with hepatic impairment may have a higher risk of developing renal insufficiency<br>• Patients should be informed of the need for regular laboratory monitoring<br>• Pregnancy Category C |
| **Adverse Events** | • Tremor<br>• Headache<br>• Diarrhea<br>• Hypertension<br>• Nausea<br>• Renal dysfunction |
| **Drug Interactions** | *Drugs with Synergistic Nephrotoxicity*<br>• Gentamicin<br>• Tobramycin<br>• Vancomycin<br>• TMP-SMX<br>• Cimetidine<br>• Ranitidine<br>• Amphotericin B<br>• Ketoconazole<br>• Melphalan<br>• Diclofenac<br>• Azapropazon<br><br>*Drugs that Increase Tacrolimus Levels*<br>• Diltiazem<br>• Nicardipine<br>• Verapamil<br>• Ketoconazole<br>• Fluconazole<br>• Itraconazole<br>• Erythromycin<br>• Clarithromycin<br>• Cimetidine<br>• Danazol<br>• Bromocriptine<br>• Methylprednisolone<br>• Metoclopramide<br>• Cyclosporine |

*Continued ...*

# Tacrolimus (FK-506)

| | |
|---|---|
| **Drug Interactions** (continued) | *Drugs that Decrease Tacrolimus Levels*<br>• Rifampin • Carbamazepine<br>• Rifabutin • Phenobarbitol<br>• Phenytoin<br><br>*Other*<br>• Vaccinations—live vaccinations should be avoided |
| **Formulations** | • 1 mg capsules supplied in 100 count bottles<br>• 5 mg capsules supplied in 100 count bottles<br>• 1 mL ampules containing the equivalent of 5 mg of anhydrous tacrolimus per mL—supplied in boxes of 10 ampules |
| **Dosage and Administration** | *IV Infusion*<br>• 0.05 mg/kg/d to 0.10 mg/kg/d administered no sooner than 6 hours after transplantation<br>• Patients should be converted to oral therapy as soon as can be tolerated<br><br>*Capsules*<br>• 0.15 mg/kg/d to 0.30 mg/kg/d administered in 2 divided daily doses every 12 hours<br>• First dose should be given 8 to 12 hours after discontinuing IV infusion |

*Editors' Notes:*

Tacrolimus appears to be a more effective drug than cyclosporine for liver transplantation. Rescue for refractory liver and kidney rejection has also been shown to be an important use for the drug. Studies in renal transplant recipients have recently been completed.

# Investigational Agents

## Rapamycin (sirolimus)

| | |
|---|---|
| **Brand Name** | Rapamune |
| **Company** | Wyeth-Ayerst Laboratories |
| **Class** | • Macrolide antibiotic with immunosuppressant properties |
| **Mechanism of Action** | • Forms a complex with FK binding proteins, inhibiting lymphocyte effects driven by certain cytokine receptors, particularly interleukin-2 |
| **Potential Applications** | • Prevention and treatment of allograft rejection |
| **Reported Adverse Events** | • Myocardial necrosis and vascular damage have been reported in animal studies |

# 15-Deoxyspergualin

| | |
|---|---|
| **Other Name** | Gusperimus |
| **Company** | Bristol-Myers Squibb Company |
| **Class** | • Antibiotic with immunosuppressant properties |
| **Mechanism of Action** | • Exact mechanism is unknown, however, it has been observed to suppress macrophage function and antigen presentation and to affect lymphocytes |
| **Potential Application** | • Rescue agent for allograft rejection |
| **Reported Adverse Events** | • Perioral numbness<br>• Feeling of facial warmth<br>• Gastrointestinal problems<br>• Fatigue<br>• Dull headache |

# Chapter 2
# Antimicrobials

## Antivirals Overview

- Acyclovir
- Famciclovir
- Ganciclovir
- Immunoglobulin
- CMV Hyperimmune Globulin
- Foscarnet Sodium

## Antibiotics Overview

- TMP-SMX
- Penicillins with Beta-Lactamase Inhibitor
- Ofloxacin
- Ciprofloxacin
- Cephalosporins
- Aminoglycosides

## Antifungals Overview

- Nystatin Suspension
- Clotrimazole Troche
- Fluconazole
- Amphotericin B
- Amphotericin B Lipid Complex Injection
- Miconazole Vaginal Cream 2%
- Ketoconazole

# Antivirals Overview

| Agent | Dosage |
| --- | --- |
| **Acyclovir** | *Mucosal and Cutaneous HSV Infection in Immunocompromised Patients*<br>• In adults, 5 mg/kg IV infused at a constant rate over 1 hour, every 8 hours (15 mg/kg/d IV) for 7 days<br>• In children under 12 years of age, 250 $mg/m^2$ IV at a constant rate over 1 hour, every 8 hours (750 $mg/m^2/d$ IV) for 7 days<br><br>*HSV Encephalitis*<br>• In adults, 10 mg/kg IV infused at a constant rate over 1 hour, every 8 hours (30 mg/kg/d IV) for 10 days<br>• In children between 6 months and 12 years of age, 500 $mg/m^2$ IV at a constant rate over 1 hour, every 8 hours (1500 $mg/m^2/d$ IV) for 10 days<br><br>*Varicella Zoster Infection in Immunocompromised Patients*<br>• In adults, 10 mg/kg IV infused at a constant rate over 1 hour, every 8 hours (30 mg/kg/d IV) for 7 days<br>• In children under 12 years of age, 500 $mg/m^2$ IV at a constant rate over 1 hour, every 8 hours (1500 $mg/m^2/d$ IV) for 7 days |
| **Famciclovir** | • 500 mg every 8 hours for 7 days |
| **Ganciclovir** | • 5 mg/kg IV given at a constant rate over 1 hour every 12 hours for 7 to 14 days<br>• Followed by 5 mg/kg/d IV on 7 days each week, or 6 mg/kg/d on 5 days each week<br>• Duration of therapy depends on degree of immunosuppression; in clinical trials, treatment was continued until postop day 100 to 120 |
| **Immunoglobulin** | • 400 mg/kg for 2 to 5 days or 800 mg/kg for 2 days |
| **CMV Hyperimmune Globulin** | • 150 mg/kg within 72 hours of transplantation<br>• 100 mg/kg at 2, 4, 6, and 8 weeks posttransplant<br>• 50 mg/kg at 12 and 16 weeks posttransplant |
| **Foscarnet Sodium** | *Induction—Normal Renal Function*<br>• 60 mg/kg IV at a constant rate over a minimum of 1 hour every 8 hours for 2 to 3 weeks depending on clinical response<br><br>*Maintenance—Normal Renal Function*<br>• 90 mg/kg/d to 120 mg/kg/d IV infused over 2 hours |

# Acyclovir

| | |
|---|---|
| **Brand Name** | Zovirax® |
| **Company** | Glaxo Wellcome Inc. |
| **Class** | Synthetic nucleoside analogue with antiviral properties against herpesviruses |
| **Mechanism of Action** | • Interferes with DNA polymerase of herpesvirus cells, inhibiting their replication |
| **Indications** | • Treatment of initial and recurrent mucosal and cutaneous herpes simplex virus (HSV-1 & HSV-2) in immunocompromised patients<br>• Treatment of herpes simplex virus encephalitis<br>• Treatment of varicella zoster virus infection in immunocompromised patients |
| **Contraindication** | • Hypersensitivity to acyclovir |
| **Warning** | • Acyclovir sodium is intended only for intravenous infusion, which should be given over a period of 1 hour to reduce the risk of renal tubular damage |
| **Special Precautions** | • Recommended dosage, frequency, and length of treatment should not be exceeded<br>• Precipitation of acyclovir crystals in renal tubules can occur, potentially leading to renal tubular damage<br>• Dosage adjustments should be based on estimated creatinine clearance<br>• 1% of patients have experienced encephalopathic changes<br>• Resistant strains have developed after repeated exposure to acyclovir<br>• Pregnancy Category C |
| **Adverse Reactions** | • Inflammation or phlebitis at injection site<br>• Transient elevations in serum creatinine and BUN<br>• Nausea and/or vomiting<br>• Itching, rash, or hives<br>• Elevation of transaminases<br>• Encephalopathic changes, including lethargy, obtundation, tremors, confusion, hallucinations, agitation, seizures, and coma |
| **Drug Interaction** | • Probenecid |
| **Formulations** | • 10 mL vial containing 500 mg<br>• 20 mL vial containing 1000 mg<br>• Also available in ointment, capsules, tablets, and suspension formulations |
| **Dosage** | Caution: Rapid or bolus intravenous and intramuscular or subcutaneous injection must be avoided<br><br>*Mucosal and Cutaneous HSV Infection in Immunocompromised Patients*<br>• In adults, 5 mg/kg IV infused at a constant rate over 1 hour, every 8 hours (15 mg/kg/d IV) for 7 days<br>• In children under 12 years of age, 250 mg/$m^2$ IV at a constant rate over 1 hour, every 8 hours (750 mg/$m^2$/d IV) for 7 days<br><br>*HSV Encephalitis*<br>• In adults, 10 mg/kg IV infused at a constant rate over 1 hour, every 8 hours (30 mg/kg/d IV) for 10 days<br>• In children between 6 months and 12 years of age, 500 mg/$m^2$ IV at a constant rate over 1 hour, every 8 hours (1500 mg/$m^2$/d IV) for 10 days |

*Continued ...*

# Acyclovir

**Dosage**

*Varicella Zoster Infection in Immunocompromised Patients*

- In adults, 10 mg/kg IV infused at a constant rate over 1 hour, every 8 hours (30 mg/kg/d IV) for 7 days
- In children under 12 years of age, 500 mg/m$^2$ IV at a constant rate over 1 hour, every 8 hours (1500 mg/m$^2$/d IV) for 7 days

*Dosing Adjustments for Patients With Renal Dysfunction*

| Creatinine clearance (mL/min/1.73m$^2$) | % of recommended dose | Dosing interval (hrs) |
|---|---|---|
| >50 | 100% | 8 |
| 25 to 50 | 100% | 12 |
| 10 to 25 | 100% | 24 |
| 0 to 10 | 50% | 24 |

*Editors' Notes:*

Very effective for prevention of herpes simplex. Many centers use high-dose acyclovir to prevent CMV infection, but studies conflict as to its effectiveness. Valacyclovir, a new antiviral, is contraindicated in immunocompromised patients due to reported cases of hemolytic anemic syndrome in transplant recipients.

# Famciclovir

| | |
|---|---|
| **Brand Name** | Famvir® |
| **Company** | SmithKline Beecham Pharmaceuticals |
| **Class** | Synthetic acyclic guanine derivative |
| **Mechanism of Action** | • Inhibits HSV-2 polymerase competitively with deoxyguanosine triphosphate, selectively inhibiting herpes viral DNA synthesis and replication |
| **Indication** | • Management of acute herpes zoster |
| **Contraindication** | • Hypersensitivity to famciclovir |
| **Precautions** | • Efficacy has not been studied in ophthalmic zoster, disseminated zoster, or in immunocompromised patients<br>• Dosage adjustment is recommended in patients with creatinine clearance values <60 mL/min<br>• Teratogenic effects—Pregnancy Category B |
| **Adverse Reactions** | • Headache<br>• Nausea<br>• Fatigue |
| **Drug Interactions** | • Cimetidine<br>• Allopurinol<br>• Theophylline<br>• Digoxin |
| **Formulation** | • 500 mg film-coated tablets in bottles of 30 and in Single-Unit Packages of 50 |
| **Dosage** | • 500 mg every 8 hours for 7 days |

*Dosing Adjustments for Patients with Renal Dysfunction*

| Creatinine Clearance (mL/min) | Dosing Regimen |
|---|---|
| ≥60 | 500 mg every 8 hours |
| 40 to 59 | 500 mg every 12 hours |
| 20 to 39 | 500 mg every 24 hours |

*Editors' Notes:*

Little data in transplant patients has been generated. There is some data regarding famciclovir for treatment of recurrent hepatitis B following liver transplantation.

# Ganciclovir

| | |
|---|---|
| **Brand Name** | Cytovene® |
| **Company** | Roche Laboratories |
| **Class** | Synthetic nucleoside analogue with antiviral properties against herpesviruses |
| **Mechanism of Action** | • Inhibits replication of herpesvirus by interfering with cellular DNA |
| **Indication** | • Prevention of CMV disease in transplant recipients at risk for CMV disease |
| **Contraindication** | • Hypersensitivity to ganciclovir or acyclovir |
| **Warnings** | • Should not be administered if the absolute neutrophil count is <500 cells/mm³ or the platelet count is <25,000 cells/mm³<br>• Should be used with caution in patients with pre-existing cytopenias or a history of cytopenic reactions to other agents or procedures<br>• May impair fertility<br>• Because of the mutagenic potential of ganciclovir, women of childbearing age should use effective contraception |
| **Special Precautions** | • Exceeding recommended dosage and infusion rate could result in increased toxicity<br>• Dosage adjustment is required in presence of renal impairment<br>• Phlebitis and pain may occur at injection site |
| **Adverse Reactions** | • Granulocytopenia<br>• Thrombocytopenia<br>• Transient elevations in serum creatinine<br>• Headache and confusion<br>• Sepsis<br>• Anemia<br>• Fever<br>• Rash<br>• Abnormal liver function values |
| **Drug Interactions** | • Probenecid<br>• Dapsone<br>• Pentamidine<br>• Flucytosine<br>• Vincristine<br>• Vinblastine<br>• Adriamycin<br>• Amphotericin B<br>• TMP-SMX<br>• Other nucleoside analogues<br>• Cyclosporine |
| **Formulation** | • 10 mL vial containing 500 mg |

*Continued ...*

# Ganciclovir

**Dosage**

- 5 mg/kg IV given at a constant rate over 1 hour every 12 hours for 7 to 14 days
- Followed by 5 mg/kg/d IV on 7 days each week, or 6 mg/kg/d on 5 days each week
- Duration of therapy depends on degree of immunosuppression; in clinical trials, treatment was continued until postop day 100 to 120

*Dosing Adjustments for Patients with Renal Dysfunction*

| Creatinine clearance (mL/min) | Induction dose (mg/kg) | Dosing interval (hrs) | Maintenance dose (mg/kg) | Dosing interval (hrs) |
|---|---|---|---|---|
| ≥70 | 5.0 | 12 | 5.0 | 24 |
| 50 to 69 | 2.5 | 12 | 2.5 | 24 |
| 25 to 49 | 2.5 | 24 | 1.25 | 24 |
| 10 to 24 | 1.25 | 24 | 0.625 | 24 |
| <10 | 1.25 | 3x/week following hemodialysis | 0.625 | 3x/week following hemodialysis |

*Editors' Notes:*

Recent data suggest that ganciclovir can decrease CMV disease when given prophylactically during OKT3 or ATG treatment. Duration of therapy for CMV at our center is as follows:

- CMV syndrome: 7 to 10 days
- CMV infection (i.e., positive blood culture): 10 to 14 days
- CMV disease: 14 to 28 days

More effective in vitro against Epstein-Barr virus than acyclovir.

# Immunoglobulin

| | |
|---|---|
| **Brand Name/ Company** | • Gammagard®/Baxter Healthcare Corporation<br>• Gamimune®N/Bayer Corporation<br>• Sandoglobulin®/Novartis |
| **Class** | • Antibody product containing in concentrated form all IgG antibodies that regularly occur in the donor population |
| **Mechanism of Action** | • Preparations contain IgG anti-CMV antibodies that neutralize CMV |
| **Application in Transplantation** | • CMV prophylaxis and treatment |
| **Contraindications** | • Hypersensitivity to human immunoglobulin<br>• Selective IgA deficiency |
| **Warnings** | • Should be administered intravenously; other routes have not been investigated<br>• Rate of infusion may cause a precipitous fall in blood pressure and a clinical picture of anaphylaxis even in the absence of hypersensitivity |
| **Special Precaution** | • Pregnancy Category C |
| **Adverse Reactions** | • Headache<br>• Fatigue<br>• Chills<br>• Backaches<br>• Leg cramps<br>• Lightheadedness<br>• Fever<br>• Urticaria<br>• Flushing<br>• Slight elevations in blood pressure<br>• Nausea/vomiting |
| **Drug Interactions** | • Drug interactions have not been evaluated. However, it is recommended that immunoglobulin be administered separately from other agents |
| **Formulations** | • 0.5 g single use bottle<br>• 1 g vial<br>• 2.5 g single use bottle<br>• 3 g vial<br>• 5.0 g single use bottle<br>• 6 g vial<br>• 10.0 g single use bottle<br>• 10 mL<br>• 50 mL<br>• 100 mL<br>• 250 mL |
| **Dosage** | • 400 mg/kg for 2 to 5 days or 800 mg/kg for 2 days |

*Editors' Notes:*

Effective at preventing CMV disease but more expensive than prophylactic ganciclovir. The cost and limited effectiveness of these products do not justify their continued use in transplant patients.

# CMV Hyperimmune Globulin

| | |
|---|---|
| **Brand Name** | CytoGam® |
| **Company** | MedImmune, Inc. |
| **Class** | • Immunoglobulin G preparation with antiviral properties |
| **Mechanism of Action** | • Contains a high concentration of IgG antibodies directed at CMV and, in individuals exposed to CMV, can elevate CMV-specific antibodies to levels sufficient to attenuate incidence of serious CMV disease |
| **Indication** | • Attenuation of primary CMV infection associated with renal transplantation in recipients who are CMV-negative and receive an organ from a CMV-positive donor |
| **Contraindications** | • Hypersensitivity to human immunoglobulin preparations<br>• Selective IgA deficiency |
| **Warning** | • During administration, patients' vital signs should be monitored closely and epinephrine should be available for treatment of an acute anaphylactic reaction |
| **Special Precautions** | • If hypotension or anaphylaxis occurs, treatment should be discontinued immediately<br>• Does not contain a preservative and, accordingly, the vial should be entered only once after reconstitution<br>• Pregnancy Category C |
| **Adverse Reactions** | • Flushing<br>• Chills<br>• Muscle cramps<br>• Back pain<br>• Fever<br>• Nausea/vomiting<br>• Wheezing |
| **Drug Interactions** | • May interfere with the immune response to live virus vaccines<br>• Drug interactions have not been evaluated. However, it is recommended that immunoglobulin be administered separately from other agents |
| **Formulation** | • Single dose vial containing 2500 mg ± 250 mg of lyophilized immunoglobulin for reconstitution with 50 mL of Sterile Water for Injection |
| **Dosage** | • 150 mg/kg within 72 hours of transplantation<br>• 100 mg/kg at 2, 4, 6, and 8 weeks posttransplant<br>• 50 mg/kg at 12 and 16 weeks posttransplant |

*Editors' Notes:*

Effective at preventing CMV disease, but more expensive than prophylactic ganciclovir. May also be useful as adjunctive therapy to ganciclovir in CMV disease.

# Foscarnet Sodium

| | |
|---|---|
| **Brand Name** | Foscavir® |
| **Company** | Astra USA, Inc. |
| **Class** | • Organic analogue of inorganic pyrophosphate that inhibits replication of all known herpesviruses in vitro |
| **Mechanism of Action** | • Selective inhibition at the pyrophosphate binding site on virus-specific DNA polymerases and reverse transcriptases |
| **Indication** | • Treatment of CMV retinitis in patients with AIDS |
| **Contraindication** | • Hypersensitivity to foscarnet sodium |
| **Warnings** | • Renal impairment is the major toxicity of foscarnet and it occurs to some degree in most patients<br>• Dose adjustments are necessary for patients with baseline renal dysfunction and in patients who experience changes in renal function during therapy<br>• Changes in serum electrolytes may occur<br>• Neurotoxicity and seizures have been reported in association with foscarnet therapy |
| **Special Precautions** | • Should be administered at recommended doses and infusion rates<br>• Anemia may occur during therapy<br>• Pregnancy Category C |
| **Adverse Reactions** | • Fever<br>• Nausea<br>• Anemia<br>• Diarrhea<br>• Abnormal renal function, including acute renal failure, decreased serum creatinine clearance, and increased serum creatinine<br>• Vomiting<br>• Headache<br>• Seizure |
| **Drug Interactions** | • Pentamidine<br>• Drugs that impair renal tubular secretions (aminoglycosides, amphotericin B)<br>• Drugs known to affect serum calcium levels |
| **Formulations** | • 24 mg/mL in 250 mL bottle<br>• 24 mg/mL in 500 mL bottle |

*Continued ...*

# Foscarnet Sodium

**Dosage**

Rate of infusion must be carefully controlled with infusion pump

*Induction—Normal Renal Function*

- 60 mg/kg IV at a constant rate over a minimum of 1 hour every 8 hours for 2 to 3 weeks depending on clinical response

*Maintenance—Normal Renal Function*

- 90 mg/kg/d to 120 mg/kg/d IV infused over 2 hours

*Dose Adjustments—Impaired Renal Function*

Induction

| CrCl (mL/min/kg) | Equivalent to 60 mg/kg q8h |
|---|---|
| ≥1.6 | 60 |
| 1.5 | 57 |
| 1.4 | 53 |
| 1.3 | 49 |
| 1.2 | 46 |
| 1.1 | 42 |
| 1.0 | 39 |
| 0.9 | 35 |
| 0.8 | 32 |
| 0.7 | 28 |
| 0.6 | 25 |
| 0.5 | 21 |
| 0.4 | 18 |

Maintenance

| CrCl (mL/min/kg) | Equivalent to 90 mg/kg/d | Equivalent to 120 mg/kg/d |
|---|---|---|
| ≥1.4 | 90 | 120 |
| 1.2 to 1.4 | 78 | 104 |
| 1.0 to 1.2 | 75 | 100 |
| 0.8 to 1.0 | 71 | 94 |
| 0.6 to 0.8 | 63 | 84 |
| 0.4 to 0.6 | 57 | 76 |

# Antibiotics Overview

| Agent | Dosage |
|---|---|
| **TMP-SMX** | *IV Infusion*<br>• *Pneumocystis carinii* pneumonia—15 mg/kg/d to 20 mg/kg/d given in 3 or 4 equally divided doses every 6 to 8 hours for up to 14 days<br>• UTI/Shigellosis—8 mg/kg/d to 10 mg/kg/d given in 2 or 4 equally divided doses every 6, 8, or 12 hours for up to 14 days for severe UTIs and for 5 days for shigellosis<br><br>*Tablets*<br>• *Pneumocystis carinii* pneumonia—15 mg/kg/d to 20 mg/kg/d TMP and 75 mg/kg/d to 100 mg/kg/d SMX in equally divided doses every 6 hours for 14 to 21 days<br>• Chronic bronchitis—2 tablets every 12 hours for 14 days<br>• Travelers' diarrhea—2 tablets every 12 hours for 5 days<br>• UTI/Shigellosis—2 tablets every 12 hours for 10 to 14 days for UTIs and for 5 days for shigellosis<br>• Otitis media (children)—8 mg/kg/d TMP and 40 mg/kg/d SMX given in 2 equally divided doses every 12 hours for 10 days |
| **Penicillins with Beta-Lactamase Inhibitor** | *Amoxicillin/Clavulanate potassium*<br>• One 250 mg tablet every 8 hours<br>• One 500 mg tablet every 8 hours for serious infection<br><br>*Ticarcillin/Clavulanate potassium*<br>• 3.1 g vial every 4 to 6 hours for systemic and urinary tract infections<br>• 200 mg/kg/d in divided doses every 6 hours for moderate gynecologic infections<br>• 300 mg/kg/d in divided doses every 4 hours for severe gynecologic infections |
| **Ofloxacin** | *Tablets*<br>• 200 mg to 400 mg every 12 hours<br>• Duration of therapy varies from 1 day for gonorrhea, to 3 days for cystitis due to *E. coli* or *K. pneumoniae*, to 7 days for UTIs and other sexually transmitted diseases, to 10 days for lower respiratory tract and skin and skin structure infections, and to 6 weeks for prostatitis<br><br>*IV Infusion*<br>• 200 mg to 400 mg by slow infusion over 60 minutes every 12 hours<br>• Duration of therapy varies from 1 day for gonorrhea, to 3 days for cystitis due to *E. coli* or *K. pneumoniae*, to 7 days for UTIs and other sexually transmitted diseases, to 10 days for lower respiratory tract and skin and skin structure infections, and to 6 weeks for prostatitis |
| **Ciprofloxacin** | *Tablets*<br>• 250 mg every 12 hours for urinary tract infection; patients with complicated infections may require 500 mg every 12 hours<br>• A single 250 mg dose for urethral and cervical gonococcal infections<br>• 500 mg every 12 hours for lower respiratory infection, skin and skin structure infection, infectious diarrhea, and bone and joint infection; serious infection may require 750 mg every 12 hours<br>• Duration of therapy is usually 7 to 14 days; bone and joint infections may require therapy for 4 to 6 weeks; infectious diarrhea may be treated for 5 to 7 days |

*Continued ...*

# Antibiotics Overview

| | |
|---|---|
| **Ciprofloxacin** (continued) | *IV Infusion*<br>• 200 mg every 12 hours for mild to moderate urinary tract infections; 400 mg every 12 hours for severe urinary tract infections<br>• 400 mg every 12 hours for lower respiratory infection, skin and skin structure infection, and bone and joint infection<br>• Duration of therapy is usually 7 to 14 days; bone and joint infections may require therapy for 4 to 6 weeks |
| **Cephalosporins** | *Cefazolin*<br>• Treatment<br>  • moderate/severe: 500 mg to 1 g every 6 to 8 hours<br>  • mild: 250 mg to 500 mg every 8 hours<br>  • UTIs: 1 g every 12 hours<br>  • Pneumonia: 500 mg every 12 hours<br>  • Severe/life-threatening: 1 g to 1.5 g every 6 hours<br>• Prophylaxis: 1 g IV or IM administered once 30 to 60 minutes prior to surgery; 500 mg to 1 g IV or IM may be given intraoperatively during lengthy procedures; 500 mg to 1 g IV or IM every 6 to 8 hours for 24 hours postop<br><br>*Cefotetan*<br>• Treatment: 1 g or 2 g IV or IM every 12 hours for 5 to 10 days<br>• Prophylaxis: 1 g or 2 g IV administered once 30 to 60 minutes prior to surgery |
| **Aminoglycosides** | *Amikacin—Patients with Normal Renal Function*<br>• 15 mg/kg/d IM or IV divided into 2 or 3 equal doses administered at equally divided intervals<br>• Usual duration of treatment is 7 to 10 days and it is desirable to limit the duration to the shortest time possible<br><br>*Tobramycin/Gentamicin—Patients with Normal Renal Function*<br>• 3 mg/kg/d IM or IV divided into 3 equal doses every 8 hours<br>• Patients with life-threatening infections may be given up to 5 mg/kg/d in 3 or 4 equal doses, with a reduction to 3 mg/kg/d as soon as clinically indicated<br>• Usual duration of treatment is 7 to 10 days and it is desirable to limit the duration to the shortest time possible |

# Trimethoprim and Sulfamethoxazole (TMP-SMX)

| | |
|---|---|
| **Brand Name/ Company** | • Septra®/Glaxo Wellcome Inc.<br>• Bactrim™/Roche Laboratories |
| **Class** | • Synthetic antibacterial combinations with activity against *Escherichia coli, Proteus* species, *Morganella morganii, Proteus mirabilis, Klebsiella* species, *Enterobacter* species, *Hemophilus influenzae, Streptococcus pneumoniae, Shigella flexneri,* and *Shigella sonnei* |
| **Mechanism of Action** | • TMP-SMX blocks 2 consecutive steps in the biosynthesis of nucleic acids and proteins essential to many bacteria |
| **Indications** | *IV Infusion*<br>• Prophylaxis and treatment of *Pneumocystis carinii* pneumonia<br>• Shigellosis<br>• Severe or complicated urinary tract infections<br><br>*Tablets*<br>• Prophylaxis and treatment of *Pneumocystis carinii* pneumonia<br>• Acute exacerbation of chronic bronchitis<br>• Urinary tract infections<br>• Travelers' diarrhea in adults<br>• Shigellosis<br>• Acute otitis media |
| **Contraindications** | • Hypersensitivity to TMP or SMX<br>• Megaloblastic anemia due to folate deficiency<br>• Pregnancy at term and nursing<br>• Infants <2 months of age |
| **Warnings** | • Deaths due to following severe reactions have occurred after treatment with SMX<br>  • Stevens-Johnson syndrome<br>  • Toxic epidermal necrolysis<br>  • Fulminant hepatic necrosis<br>  • Agranulocytosis<br>  • Aplastic anemia<br>  • Other blood dyscrasias<br>  • Hypersensitivity of the respiratory tract<br>• Should not be used for the treatment of streptococcal pharyngitis |
| **Special Precautions** | • Should be given with caution to patients with renal or hepatic impairment, folate deficiency, and severe allergy or asthma<br>• Pregnancy Category C |
| **Adverse Reactions** | • Gastrointestinal disturbances (nausea, vomiting, anorexia)<br>• Allergic skin reactions (rash, urticaria)<br>• Agranulocytosis, aplastic anemia, and other blood dyscrasias<br>• Stevens-Johnson syndrome, toxic epidermal necrolysis, and other allergic reactions<br>• Hepatitis, including cholestatic jaundice and hepatic necrosis<br>• Renal failure and interstitial nephritis<br>• Aseptic meningitis, convulsions, peripheral neuritis, ataxia, vertigo, tinnitus, and headache<br>• Hallucinations, depression, apathy, and nervousness |

*Continued ...*

Immuno-suppression | Antimicrobials | Cardiovascular Agents | Antiosteo-porosis Agents | Antiplatelets | Diabetes Agents | Ulcer Treatment | Diuretics | Other Agents

# Trimethoprim and Sulfamethoxazole (TMP-SMX)

| | | |
|---|---|---|
| **Drug Interactions** | • Thiazides<br>• Warfarin<br>• Phenytoin<br>• Methotrexate<br>• Serum methotrexate assays<br>• Jaffe alkaline picrate reaction assay | |
| **Formulations** | *IV Infusion*<br>• 5 mL vial containing 80 mg TMP (16 mg/mL) and 400 mg (80 mg/mL) SMX<br>• 10 mL vial containing 160 mg (16 mg/mL) TMP and 800 mg (80 mg/mL) SMX<br>• 20 mL vial containing 320 mg (16 mg/mL) TMP and 1600 mg (80 mg/mL) SMX<br><br>*Tablets*<br>• Tablets containing 80 mg TMP and 400 mg SMX supplied in bottles of 100<br>• Double-strength tablets containing 160 mg TMP and 800 mg SMX supplied in bottles of 100 | |
| **Dosage** | *IV Infusion* | |
| | • *Pneumocystis carinii* pneumonia | 15 mg/kg/d to 20 mg/kg/d given in 3 or 4 equally divided doses every 6 to 8 hours for up to 14 days |
| | • UTI/Shigellosis | 8 mg/kg/d to 10 mg/kg/d given in 2 or 4 equally divided doses every 6, 8, or 12 hours for up to 14 days for severe UTIs and for 5 days for shigellosis |
| | *Tablets* | |
| | • *Pneumocystis carinii* pneumonia | 15 mg/kg/d to 20 mg/kg/d TMP and 75 mg/kg/d to 100 mg/kg/d SMX in equally divided doses every 6 hours for 14 to 21 days |
| | • Chronic bronchitis | 2 tablets every 12 hours for 14 days |
| | • Travelers' diarrhea | 2 tablets every 12 hours for 5 days |
| | • UTI/Shigellosis | 2 tablets every 12 hours for 10 to 14 days for UTIs and for 5 days for shigellosis |
| | • Otitis media (children) | 8 mg/kg/d TMP and 40 mg/kg/d SMX given in 2 equally divided doses every 12 hours for 10 days |

*Editors' Notes:*

**Best randomized trials:**

Fox BC, Sollinger HW, Belzer FO, Maki DG. A prospective, randomized, double-blind study of trimethoprim-sulfamethoxazole for prophylaxis of infection in renal transplantation: clinical efficacy, absorption of trimethoprim-sulfamethoxazole, effects on the microflora, and the cost-benefit of prophylaxis. *Am J Med.* 1990; 89:225-274.

Maki DG, Fox BC, Gould JR, Sollinger HW, Belzer FO. A prospective, randomized, double-blind study of trimethoprim-sulfamethoxazole for prophylaxis of infection in renal transplantation: side effects of trimethoprim-sulfamethoxazole, interaction with cyclosporine-A. *J Lab Clin Med.* 1992; 119(1):11-24.

# Penicillins With Beta-Lactamase Inhibitor

| | |
|---|---|
| **Brand Name** | • Augmentin® (amoxicillin/clavulanate potassium)<br>• Timentin® (ticarcillin/clavulanate potassium) |
| **Company** | • SmithKline Beecham Pharmaceuticals |
| **Class** | • Synthetic antibacterial combinations containing a penicillin (amoxicillin/ticarcillin) and a beta-lactamase inhibitor<br>• Both have activity against *Staphylococcus aureus, Staphylococcus epidermidis, Staphylococcus saprophyticus, Streptococcus faecalis, Streptococcus pneumoniae, Streptococcus pyogenes, Streptococcus viridans, Clostridium* species, *Peptococcus* species, *Hemophilus influenzae, Moraxella catarrhalis, Escherichia coli, Klebsiella* species, *Enterobacter* species, *Proteus mirabilis, Proteus vulgaris, Neisseria gonorrhoeae, Legionella* species, and *Bacteroides species*<br>• Ticarcillin/Clavulanate potassium also has activity against *Pseudomonas* species, *Providencia rettgeri, Providencia stuartii, Morganella morganii, Acinetobacter* species, *Serratia* species, *Neisseria meningitidis, Salmonella* species, *Citrobacter* species, *Streptococcus bovis,* and *Streptococcus agalactiae* |
| **Mechanism of Action** | • Clavulanic acid protects penicillins from degradation by inactivating a wide range of beta-lactamase enzymes |
| **Indications** | *Amoxicillin/Clavulanate potassium*<br>• Lower respiratory infection<br>• Otitis media<br>• Sinusitis<br>• Skin and skin structure infection<br>• Urinary tract infection<br><br>*Ticarcillin/Clavulanate potassium*<br>• Septicemia<br>• Lower respiratory infection<br>• Bone and joint infection<br>• Skin and skin structure infection<br>• Urinary tract infection<br>• Gynecologic infection<br>• Intra-abdominal infection |
| **Contraindication** | • History of allergic reactions to penicillins |
| **Warnings** | • Serious and occasionally fatal anaphylactoid reactions have been reported in patients on penicillin therapy<br>• Serious anaphylactoid reactions require immediate emergency treatment with epinephrine<br>• Pseudomembranous colitis has been reported |
| **Special Precautions** | • Superinfections with mycotic or bacterial pathogens may occur<br>• Pregnancy Category B |

*Continued ...*

# Penicillins With Beta-Lactamase Inhibitor

| | |
|---|---|
| **Adverse Reactions** | • Skin rash, pruritus, urticaria, arthralgia, myalgia, drug fever, chills, chest discomfort, anaphylactic reactions<br>• Headache, giddiness, neuromuscular hyperirritability, convulsive seizures<br>• Taste and smell disturbances, stomatitis, flatulence, nausea, vomiting, diarrhea, epigastric pain, pseudomembranous colitis<br>• Thrombocytopenia, leukopenia, neutropenia, reduction of hematocrit and hemoglobin<br>• Abnormal hepatic and renal function tests<br>• Pain, burning, swelling, and induration at injection site |
| **Drug Interactions** | • Aminoglycosides<br>• Probenecid<br>• False-positive protein reactions<br>• False-positive Coombs' test |
| **Formulations** | *Amoxicillin/Clavulanate potassium*<br>• 250 mg tablets (250 mg amoxicillin/125 mg clavulanic acid)<br>• 500 mg tablets (500 mg amoxicillin/125 mg clavulanic acid)<br>• 125 mg/5 mL for oral suspension (125 mg amoxicillin/31.25 mg clavulanic acid)<br>• 250 mg/5 mL for oral suspension (250 mg amoxicillin/62.5 mg clavulanic acid)<br>• 125 mg chewable tablets (125 mg amoxicillin/31.25 mg clavulanic acid)<br>• 250 mg chewable tablets (250 mg amoxicillin/62.5 mg clavulanic acid)<br><br>*Ticarcillin/Clavulanate potassium*<br>• 3.1 and 3.2 gram vials and Piggyback bottles |
| **Dosage** | *Amoxicillin/Clavulanate potassium*<br>• One 250 mg tablet every 8 hours<br>• One 500 mg tablet every 8 hours for serious infection<br><br>*Ticarcillin/Clavulanate potassium*<br>• 3.1 g vial every 4 to 6 hours for systemic and urinary tract infections<br>• 200 mg/kg/d in divided doses every 6 hours for moderate gynecologic infections<br>• 300 mg/kg/d in divided doses every 4 hours for severe gynecologic infections |

*Editors' Notes:*

Augmentin and Timentin are frequently used for diabetic foot infections and urinary tract infections.

# Ofloxacin

| | |
|---|---|
| **Brand Name** | Floxin® |
| **Company** | Ortho-McNeil Pharmaceutical |
| **Class** | • Synthetic, broad-spectrum quinolone with activity against *Chlamydia trachomatis, Chlamydia pneumoniae, Escherichia coli, Klebsiella pneumoniae, Klebsiella oxytoca, Enterobacter aerogenes, Enterobacter cloacae, Citrobacter diversus, Citrobacter freundii, Proteus mirabilis, Proteus vulgaris, Providencia stuartii, Providencia rettgeri, Morganella morganii, Serratia marcescens, Pseudomonas aeruginosa, Acinetobacter calcoaceticus, Bordetella parapertussis, Bordetella pertussis, Haemophilus influenzae, Haemophilus ducreyi, Neisseria gonorrhoeae, Neisseria meningitidis, Pseudomonas fluorescens, Moraxella catarrhalis, Campylobacter jejuni, Aeromonas hydrophila, Enterococcus faecalis, Staphylococcus aureus, Staphylococcus epidermidis, Staphylococcus saprophyticus, Streptococcus agalactiae, Streptococcus aureus, Streptococcus pneumoniae, Streptococcus pyogenes, Bacteroides fragilis, Bacteroides intermedius, Clostridium perfringens, Clostridium welchii, Eikenella corrodens, Gardnerella vaginalis, Peptococcus niger, Peptostreptococcus* species, *Legionella pneumophila, Mycobacterium tuberculosis, Mycoplasma hominis, Mycoplasma pneumoniae, Ureaplasma urealyticum* |
| **Mechanism of Action** | • Interferes with DNA gyrase, an enzyme that is needed for bacterial synthesis |
| **Indications** | • Lower respiratory infection<br>• Skin and skin structure infection<br>• Sexually transmitted diseases<br>• Urinary tract infection<br>• Prostate infection due to *E. coli* |
| **Contraindication** | • History of hypersensitivity to ofloxacin and other quinolones |
| **Warnings** | • Safety and efficacy of ofloxacin has not been established in children, adolescents, pregnant women, and lactating women<br>• Osteochondrosis has been noted in immature rats exposed to 5 to 16 times the recommended human dose<br>• Has not been shown to be effective in treating syphilis<br>• Serious hypersensitivity reactions have occurred<br>• Convulsions, increased intracranial pressure, and toxic psychosis have been reported in patients treated with quinolones<br>• Pseudomembranous colitis has been reported |
| **Special Precautions** | • Adequate hydration is required to prevent highly concentrated urine<br>• Phototoxicity has occurred after exposure to direct sunlight<br>• Should be used with caution in patients with known CNS disorders<br>• Disturbances of blood glucose have been reported—usually in diabetic patients receiving concomitant treatment with oral hypoglycemic agent<br>• Pregnancy Category C |

*Continued ...*

# Ofloxacin

| | |
|---|---|
| **Adverse Reactions** | • Nausea<br>• Insomnia<br>• Headache<br>• Dizziness<br>• Diarrhea<br>• Vomiting<br>• Rash<br>• Pruritus<br>• External genital pruritus in women<br>• Vaginitis<br>• Dysgeusia |
| **Drug Interactions** | • Nonsteroidal anti-inflammatory drugs<br>• Probenecid<br>• Theophylline<br>• Warfarin<br>• Antidiabetic agents |
| **Formulations** | • 200 mg tablets<br>• 300 mg tablets<br>• 400 mg tablets<br>• 10 mL single-use vials<br>• 20 mL single-use vials<br>• 100 mL premixed in bottles, containing the equivalent of 400 mg ofloxacin in 5% dextrose<br>• 50 mL premixed in flexible containers containing the equivalent of 200 mg ofloxacin in 5% dextrose<br>• 100 mL premixed in flexible containers containing the equivalent of 400 mg ofloxacin in 5% dextrose |
| **Dosage** | *Tablets*<br>• 200 mg to 400 mg every 12 hours<br>• Duration of therapy varies from 1 day for gonorrhea, to 3 days for cystitis due to *E. coli* or *K. pneumoniae*, to 7 days for UTIs and other sexually transmitted diseases, to 10 days for lower respiratory tract and skin and skin structure infections, and to 6 weeks for prostatitis<br><br>*IV Infusion*<br>• 200 mg to 400 mg by slow infusion over 60 minutes every 12 hours<br>• Duration of therapy varies from 1 day for gonorrhea, to 3 days for cystitis due to *E. coli* or *K. pneumoniae*, to 7 days for UTIs and other sexually transmitted diseases, to 10 days for lower respiratory tract and skin and skin structure infections, and to 6 weeks for prostatitis |

# Ciprofloxacin

| | |
|---|---|
| **Brand Name** | Cipro® |
| **Company** | Bayer Corporation |
| **Class** | • Synthetic, broad-spectrum quinolone with activity against *Escherichia coli, Klebsiella pneumoniae, Klebsiella oxytoca, Enterobacter aerogenes, Enterobacter cloacae, Citrobacter diversus, Citrobacter freundii, Edwardsiella tarda, Salmonella enteritidis, Salmonella typhi, Shigella sonnei, Shigella flexneri, Proteus mirabilis, Proteus vulgaris, Providencia stuartii, Providencia rettgeri, Morganella morganii, Serratia marcescens, Yersinia enterocolitica, Pseudomonas aeruginosa, Acinetobacter calcoaceticus* subsp. *lwoffi, Acinetobacter calcoaceticus* subsp. *anitratus, Hemophilus influenzae, Hemophilus parainfluenzae, Hemophilus ducreyi, Neisseria gonorrhoeae, Neisseria meningitidis, Moraxella catarrhalis, Campylobacter jejuni, Campylobacter coli, Aeromonas hydrophila, Aeromonas caviae, Vibrio cholerae, Vibrio parahaemolyticus, Vibrio vulnificus, Brucella melitensis, Pasteurella multocida, Legionella pneumophila, Staphylococcus* species, *Streptococcus pyogenes,* and *Streptococcus pneumoniae* |
| **Mechanism of Action** | • Interferes with DNA gyrase, an enzyme which is needed for bacterial synthesis |
| **Indications** | • Lower respiratory infection<br>• Bone and joint infection<br>• Skin and skin structure infection<br>• Urinary tract infection<br>• Infectious diarrhea |
| **Contraindication** | • History of hypersensitivity to ciprofloxacin and to other quinolones |
| **Warnings** | • Safety and efficacy of ciprofloxacin has not been established in children, adolescents, pregnant women, and lactating women<br>• Convulsions have been reported in patients receiving ciprofloxacin<br>• Serious and fatal reactions have been reported after the co-administration of ciprofloxacin and theophylline<br>• Serious hypersensitivity reactions have occurred<br>• Pseudomembranous colitis has been reported |
| **Special Precautions** | • Crystals of ciprofloxacin have been observed in urine of human subjects<br>• Phototoxicity has occurred after exposure to direct sunlight<br>• Pregnancy Category C |
| **Adverse Reactions** | • Nausea<br>• Diarrhea<br>• Vomiting<br>• Abdominal pain/discomfort<br>• Headache<br>• Restlessness<br>• Rash |

*Continued ...*

# Ciprofloxacin

| | |
|---|---|
| **Drug Interactions** | • Theophylline<br>• Caffeine<br>• Antacids containing magnesium, aluminum, or calcium<br>• Cyclosporine<br>• Warfarin<br>• Probenecid |
| **Formulations** | • Tablets containing 250 mg<br>• Capsules containing 500 mg or 750 mg<br>• 20 mL vial containing 200 mg<br>• 40 mL vial containing 400 mg<br>• 100 mL flexible container containing 200 mg<br>• 200 mL flexible container containing 400 mg |
| **Dosage** | *Tablets*<br>• 250 mg every 12 hours for urinary tract infection; patients with complicated infections may require 500 mg every 12 hours<br>• A single 250 mg dose for urethral and cervical gonococcal infections<br>• 500 mg every 12 hours for lower respiratory infection, skin and skin structure infection, infectious diarrhea, and bone and joint infection; serious infection may require 750 mg every 12 hours<br>• Duration of therapy is usually 7 to 14 days; bone and joint infections may require therapy for 4 to 6 weeks; infectious diarrhea may be treated for 5 to 7 days<br><br>*IV Infusion*<br>• 200 mg every 12 hours for mild to moderate urinary tract infections; 400 mg every 12 hours for severe urinary tract infections<br>• 400 mg every 12 hours for lower respiratory infection, skin and skin structure infection, and bone and joint infection<br>• Duration of therapy is usually 7 to 14 days; bone and joint infections may require therapy for 4 to 6 weeks |

*Editors' Notes:*

Variable effect on renal function and cyclosporine metabolism. Monitor cyclosporine levels and renal function carefully.

# Cephalosporins

| | |
|---|---|
| **Brand Name/ Company** | • Ancef® (cefazolin)/SmithKline Beecham Pharmaceuticals<br>• Cefotan® (cefotetan)/Zeneca Pharmaceuticals |
| **Class** | • Semisynthetic, broad-spectrum cephalosporin<br>• Both have activity against *Escherichia coli, Proteus mirabilis, Klebsiella* species, *Hemophilus influenzae, Staphylococcus aureus, Staphylococcus epidermidis,* and *Streptococcus pneumoniae*<br>• Cefotan also has activity against *Morganella morganii, Neisseria gonorrhoeae, Moraxella catarrhalis, Proteus vulgaris, Providencia rettgeri, Serratia marcescens, Streptococcus agalactiae, Streptococcus pyogenes, Bacteroides bivius, Bacteroides disiens, Bacteroides fragilis, Bacteroides melaninogenicus, Bacteroides vulgatus, Fusobacterium* species, and gram-positive bacilli |
| **Mechanism of Action** | • Inhibition of cell wall synthesis |
| **Indications** | • Respiratory infections<br>• Bone and joint infection<br>• Skin and skin structure infection<br>• Urinary tract infection<br>• Biliary tract infection<br>• Genital infection<br>• Septicemia<br>• Endocarditis<br>• Intra-abdominal infection<br>• Surgical prophylaxis |
| **Contraindication** | • Hypersensitivity to cephalosporin class of antibiotics |
| **Warnings** | • If patient is penicillin-sensitive, caution should be used because there have been reports of cross-hypersensitivity among beta-lactam antibiotics<br>• Pseudomembranous colitis has been reported |
| **Special Precautions** | • Patients should be monitored for signs of superinfection<br>• Pregnancy Category B |
| **Adverse Reactions** | • Diarrhea, nausea<br>• Eosinophilia, positive Coombs' test, thrombocytosis, agranulocytosis, hemolytic anemia, leukopenia, thrombocytopenia, prolonged prothrombin time<br>• Elevation of hepatic enzymes<br>• Rash, anaphylactic reaction<br>• Phlebitis at injection site |
| **Drug Interactions** | • Aminoglycosides<br>• Probenecid<br>• False-positive reaction for glucose in the urine<br>• False increases in serum and urine creatinine |

*Continued ...*

# Cephalosporins

| | | |
|---|---|---|
| **Formulations** | *Cefazolin*<br>• Vials equivalent to 500 mg or 1 g of cefazolin<br>• Piggyback Vial equivalent to 1 g of cefazolin<br>• Pharmacy Bulk Vial equivalent to 5 g or 10 g of cefazolin<br>• Frozen, sterile, nonpyrogenic solution in plastic containers equivalent to 500 mg or 1 g of cefazolin | |
| | *Cefotetan*<br>• 1 g in 10 mL vial<br>• 2 g in 20 mL vial<br>• 1 g in 100 mL vial<br>• 2 g in 100 mL vial<br>• 10 g in 100 mL vial | |
| **Dosage** | *Cefazolin* | |
| | • Treatment | |
| | • Moderate/severe | 500 mg to 1 g every 6 to 8 hours |
| | • Mild | 250 mg to 500 mg every 8 hours |
| | • UTIs | 1 g every 12 hours |
| | • Pneumonia | 500 mg every 12 hours |
| | • Severe/life-threatening | 1 g to 1.5 g every 6 hours |
| | • Prophylaxis | 1 g IV or IM administered once 30 to 60 minutes prior to surgery; 500 mg to 1 g IV or IM may be given intraoperatively during lengthy procedures; 500 mg to 1 g IV or IM every 6 to 8 hours for 24 hours postop |
| | *Cefotetan* | |
| | • Treatment | 1 g or 2 g IV or IM every 12 hours for 5 to 10 days |
| | • Prophylaxis | 1 g or 2 g IV administered once 30 to 60 minutes prior to surgery |

*Editors' Notes:*

Personal choice for prophylaxis in renal transplantation. At the University of Wisconsin, the wound infection rate after renal transplantation is 1.6%.

# Aminoglycosides

| | |
|---|---|
| **Brand Name/ Company** | • Amikin® (amikacin)/Apothecon<br>• Nebcin® (tobramycin)/Eli Lilly and Company<br>• Garamycin® (gentamicin)/Schering Corporation |
| **Class** | • Semisynthetic aminoglycoside antibiotics with activity against *Pseudomonas* species, *Escherichia coli, Proteus* species, *Providencia* species, *Klebsiella* species, *Enterobacter* species, *Serratia* species, *Acinetobacter* species, *Citrobacter freundii, Staphylococcus* species<br>• Aminoglycosides generally have a low level of activity against gram-positive organisms |
| **Mechanism of Action** | • Inhibit normal protein synthesis in susceptible organisms |
| **Indications** | • Treatment of the following serious infections due to susceptible gram-negative bacteria:<br>  • Septicemia<br>  • Respiratory tract<br>  • Bone and joint<br>  • Central nervous system<br>  • Skin and soft tissue<br>  • Intra-abdominal<br>  • Burns and postoperative infection<br>  • Complicated, recurrent UTIs (aminoglycosides are not indicated for uncomplicated, initial episodes of UTIs) |
| **Contraindication** | • History of hypersensitivity or serious toxic reaction to aminoglycosides |
| **Warnings** | • Patients should be monitored closely because of the potential for development of ototoxicity and nephrotoxicity<br>• Should be used with caution in premature and neonatal infants because of their renal immaturity<br>• Neuromuscular blockade and respiratory paralysis have been reported, and the possibility of their occurrence should be considered in patients receiving anesthetics, neuromuscular blocking agents, or in patients receiving citrate-anticoagulated blood<br>• May cause fetal damage when administered to pregnant women<br>• Bisulfite component may cause allergic reactions<br>• Concurrent use of potent diuretics should be avoided |
| **Special Precautions** | • Serum and urine specimens should be collected for periodic monitoring during therapy<br>• Pregnancy Category D<br>• Concurrent and serial use of other ototoxic, nephrotoxic, and neurotoxic agents (systemic or topical) should be avoided<br>• Increased nephrotoxicity has been reported after the concomitant use of cephalosporins<br>• Patients should be well hydrated to minimize chemical irritation of the renal tubules<br>• Dosage should be reduced if there are signs of renal dysfunction; therapy should be discontinued if azotemia increases or if there is a progressive decrease in urine output<br>• It is especially important to monitor renal function in elderly patients<br>• Should be used with caution in patients with neuromuscular disorders |

*Continued ...*

# Aminoglycosides

| | |
|---|---|
| **Adverse Reactions** | • *Neurotoxicity/Ototoxicity:* Hearing loss and/or loss of balance, dizziness, tinnitus, and roaring in the ears<br>• *Neurotoxicity/Neuromuscular blockage*: Acute muscular paralysis and apnea<br>• *Nephrotoxicity:* Elevation of serum creatinine, albuminuria, presence of red and white cells, casts, azotemia, and oliguria<br>• *Other:* Skin rash, drug fever, headache, paresthesia, tremor, nausea/vomiting, eosinophilia, arthralgia, anemia, and hypotension |
| **Drug Interactions** | • Bacitracin<br>• Cisplatin<br>• Amphotericin B<br>• Cephaloridine<br>• Paromomycin<br>• Viomycin<br>• Polymyxin B<br>• Colistin<br>• Vancomycin<br>• Other aminoglycosides<br>• Potent diuretics (ethacrynic acid)<br>• Beta-lactam antibiotics |
| **Formulations** | *Amikacin*<br>• 100 mg/2 mL vial<br>• 500 mg/2 mL vial<br>• 500 mg/2 mL disposable syringe<br>• 1 g/4 mL vial<br><br>*Gentamicin*<br>• 40 mg/mL in 2 mL vial<br>• 40 mg/mL in 1.5 mL vial<br><br>*Tobramycin*<br>• 80 mg/2 mL vial<br>• 40 mg/mL vial<br>• 20 mg/2 mL vial<br>• 60 mg/1.5 mL disposable syringe<br>• 80 mg/2 mL disposable syringe<br>• 60 mg/6 mL Add-Vantage vial<br>• 80 mg/8 mL Add-Vantage vial |
| **Dosage** | *Amikacin—Patients with Normal Renal Function*<br>• 15 mg/kg/d IM or IV divided into 2 or 3 equal doses administered at equally divided intervals<br>• Usual duration of treatment is 7 to 10 days and it is desirable to limit the duration to the shortest time possible<br><br>*Tobramycin/Gentamicin—Patients with Normal Renal Function*<br>• 3 mg/kg/d IM or IV divided into 3 equal doses every 8 hours<br>• Patients with life-threatening infections may be given up to 5 mg/kg/d in 3 or 4 equal doses, with a reduction to 3 mg/kg/d as soon as clinically indicated<br>• Usual duration of treatment is 7 to 10 days and it is desirable to limit the duration to the shortest time possible |

*Editors' Notes:*

In a septic renal transplant recipient, a loading dose of aminoglycoside may be warranted despite concerns about renal toxicity.

# Antifungals Overview

| Agent | Dosage |
|---|---|
| **Nystatin Suspension** | • 200,000 or 400,000 units 4 times a day, continued until 48 hours after symptoms have disappeared |
| **Clotrimazole Troche** | *Treatment*<br>• One troche 5 times a day for 14 consecutive days<br><br>*Prophylaxis*<br>• One troche 3 times a day until steroids are reduced to maintenance levels |
| **Fluconazole** | *Oropharyngeal Candidiasis*<br>• 200 mg on first day, followed by 100 mg/d for at least 2 weeks<br><br>*Esophageal Candidiasis*<br>• 200 mg on first day, followed by 100 mg/d for a minimum of 3 weeks and for at least 2 weeks after resolution of symptoms<br><br>*Systemic Candidiasis*<br>• Up to 400 mg/d<br><br>*Cryptococcal Meningitis*<br>• 400 mg on first day, followed by 200 mg/d for 10 to 12 weeks after cerebrospinal fluid becomes culture negative |
| **Amphotericin B** | *IV Infusion*<br>• Initially 1 mg (base) as a test dose, administered in 20 mL of 5% dextrose injection over a period of 20 to 30 minutes, with 5 mg to 10 mg incremental increases depending on patient tolerance and severity of the infection, up to a maximum of 0.5 to 0.7 mg/kg<br>• Should be infused over a period of 2 to 6 hours |
| **Amphotericin B Lipid Complex Injection** | • 5 mg/kg/d IV for invasive aspergillosis<br>• 2.0 mg/kg/d to 2.5 mg/kg/d IV for candidiasis |
| **Miconazole Vaginal Cream 2%** | *Tinea Pedis, Tinea Cruris, Tinea Corporis, and Cutaneous Candidiasis*<br>• Enough to cover affected areas twice daily (morning and evening)<br><br>*Tinea Versicolor*<br>• Enough to cover affected areas once daily |
| **Ketoconazole** | *Adults*<br>• 200 mg in a single daily administration<br>• If there is insufficient response, dose can be raised to 400 mg/d<br><br>*Children*<br>• 3.3 mg/kg to 6.6 mg/kg in a single daily dose |

# Nystatin Suspension

| | |
|---|---|
| **Brand Name/ Company** | • Mycostatin®/Bristol-Myers Oncology<br>• Generics |
| **Class** | • Antifungal with activity against *Candida albicans* and other *Candida* species |
| **Mechanism of Action** | • Binds to sterols in fungus cell membrane, resulting in an inability to function as a selective barrier and a subsequent loss of essential cellular components |
| **Indication** | • Treatment and prophylaxis of oropharyngeal candidiasis |
| **Contraindication** | • Hypersensitivity to nystatin |
| **Special Precautions** | • Patients with full or partial dentures may need to soak their dentures nightly in Mycostatin (nystatin)<br>• Pregnancy Category C |
| **Adverse Reactions** | • Diarrhea<br>• Nausea/vomiting<br>• Stomach pain |
| **Drug Interactions** | • None reported |
| **Formulations** | *Nystatin Oral Suspension*<br>• 100,000 units/mL<br><br>*Nystatin for Oral Suspension*<br>• 1,000,000,000 units/mL<br>• 2,000,000,000 units/mL<br>• One-eighth of a teaspoon equals approximately 500,000 units<br>• To prepare, one-eighth of a teaspoon of powder is added to 120 mL of water |
| **Dosage** | • 200,000 or 400,000 units 4 times a day, continued until 48 hours after symptoms have disappeared |

*Editors' Notes:*

Effective prophylaxis for oral candidiasis, especially in diabetic patients.

# Clotrimazole Troche

| | |
|---|---|
| **Brand Name** | Mycelex® |
| **Company** | Bayer Corporation |
| **Class** | • Synthetic, broad-spectrum antifungal agent with activity against *Candida albicans* and other *Candida* species |
| **Mechanism of Action** | • Inhibits growth of pathogens by altering permeability of cell membranes |
| **Indications** | • Local treatment of oropharyngeal candidiasis<br>• Prophylaxis to reduce incidence of oropharyngeal candidiasis in immunocompromised patients |
| **Contraindication** | • Hypersensitivity to clotrimazole |
| **Warning** | • Is not indicated for the treatment of systemic mycoses |
| **Special Precautions** | • Abnormal liver function tests have been reported<br>• Patients must be of age where they can understand the need to let each troche dissolve slowly in the mouth<br>• Pregnancy Category C |
| **Adverse Reactions** | • Abnormal liver function test values<br>• Nausea/vomiting<br>• Unpleasant mouth sensations<br>• Pruritus |
| **Drug Interactions** | • None reported |
| **Formulation** | • Slowly dissolving tablet containing 10 mg of clotrimazole, supplied in bottles of 70 and 140 tablets |
| **Dosage** | *Treatment*<br>• One troche 5 times a day for 14 consecutive days<br><br>*Prophylaxis*<br>• One troche 3 times a day until steroids are reduced to maintenance levels |

*Editors' Notes:*

Better compliance than with nystatin. Currently, the drug of choice for prophylaxis.

Immuno-suppression | Antimicrobials | Cardiovascular Agents | Antiosteo-porosis Agents | Antiplatelets | Diabetes Agents | Ulcer Treatment | Diuretics | Other Agents

# Fluconazole

| | |
|---|---|
| **Brand Name** | Diflucan® |
| **Company** | Roerig Division/Pfizer |
| **Class** | • Synthetic, broad-spectrum bis-triazole antifungal agent with activity against *Cryptococcus neoformans* and *Candida* species |
| **Mechanism of Action** | • Selectively inhibits fungal cytochrome P-450 sterol C-14 alpha-demethylation, leading to accumulation of 14 alpha-methyl sterols in fungi |
| **Indications** | • Treatment of oropharyngeal and esophageal candidiasis and may be effective for the treatment of serious systemic candidal infections<br>• Cryptococcal meningitis |
| **Contraindications** | • Hypersensitivity to fluconazole or to any of its excipients<br>• Caution should be used in patients with hypersensitivity to other azoles<br>• Should not be used with terfenadine or astemizole |
| **Warnings** | • Anaphylaxis has been reported<br>• Patients who develop abnormal liver function tests should be monitored for development of more serious hepatic injury<br>• Immunocompromised patients who develop rashes should be monitored closely |
| **Special Precaution** | • Pregnancy Category C |
| **Adverse Reactions** | • Nausea • Headache • Skin rash<br>• Vomiting • Abdominal pain • Diarrhea |
| **Drug Interactions** | • Increased prothrombin time after warfarin administration<br>• Phenytoin • Cyclosporine • Tolbutamide<br>• Glyburide • Glipizide • Rifampin<br>• Terfenadine • Astemizole |
| **Formulations** | • Tablets containing 50 mg, 100 mg, or 200 mg<br>• Sterile isotonic solutions containing 2 mg/mL of fluconazole in glass bottles or plastic containers holding volumes of 100 mL or 200 mL |
| **Dosage** | *Oropharyngeal Candidiasis*<br>• 200 mg on first day, followed by 100 mg/d for at least 2 weeks<br><br>*Esophageal Candidiasis*<br>• 200 mg on first day, followed by 100 mg/d for a minimum of 3 weeks and for at least 2 weeks after resolution of symptoms<br><br>*Systemic Candidiasis*<br>• Up to 400 mg/d<br><br>*Cryptococcal Meningitis*<br>• 400 mg on first day, followed by 200 mg/d for 10 to 12 weeks after cerebrospinal fluid becomes culture negative<br><br>*Dosage Adjustments for Renal Impairment* |

| CrCl (mL/min) | % of Recommended Dose |
|---|---|
| >50 | 100% |
| 11-50 | 50% |
| Patients on hemodialysis | One recommended dose after each dialysis |

***Editors' Notes:***

Commonly affects cyclosporine level. May be useful for candida UTI and esophageal candidiasis.

# Amphotericin B

| | |
|---|---|
| **Brand Name** | Fungizone® |
| **Company** | Apothecon |
| **Class** | • Antifungal polyene antibiotic obtained from a strain of *Streptomyces nodosus* |
| **Mechanism of Action** | • Binds to sterols in fungus cell membrane, resulting in an inability to function as a selective barrier and a subsequent loss of essential cellular components |
| **Indications** | • Aspergillosis<br>• Blastomycosis<br>• Candidiasis<br>• Coccidioidomycosis<br>• Cryptococcosis<br>• Endocarditis<br>• Endophthalmitis<br>• Histoplasmosis<br>• Intra-abdominal infection<br>• Leishmaniasis<br>• Meningitis (cryptococcal, fungal)<br>• Mucormycosis<br>• Septicemia<br>• Sporotrichosis<br>• Fungal urinary tract infection<br>• Meningoencephalitis<br>• Paracoccidioidomycosis |
| **Contraindications** | • Hypersensitivity to amphotericin B<br>• Renal function impairment |
| **Warning** | • Because of its toxicity, amphotericin B is indicated primarily in patients with progressive, potentially fatal infections in whom the diagnosis is firmly established, preferably by positive culture or histologic study |
| **Special Precautions** | • Pregnancy Category B<br>• It is important to monitor the following patient parameters<br>  • BUN<br>  • Serum creatinine<br>  • CBC<br>  • Platelet count<br>  • Serum magnesium and potassium |
| **Adverse Reactions** | • Anemia<br>• Hypokalemia<br>• Renal function impairment<br>• Thrombophlebitis<br>• Infusion-related illness (fever, chills, nausea, vomiting, headache, hypotension)<br>• Blurred vision<br>• Cardiac arrhythmias<br>• Hypersensitivity<br>• Leukopenia<br>• Polyneuropathy<br>• Seizures<br>• Thrombocytopenia |

*Continued ...*

# Amphotericin B

| | |
|---|---|
| **Drug Interactions** | • Adrenocorticoids, glucocorticoid, mineralocorticoid, carbonic anhydrase inhibitors, corticotropin<br>• Medications that cause blood dyscrasia or bone marrow suppression<br>• Radiation therapy<br>• Digitalis glycosides<br>• Neuromuscular blocking agents<br>• Potassium-depleting diuretics<br>• Nephrotoxic medications<br>• Flucytosine |
| **Formulation** | • 50 mg (base) |
| **Dosage** | *IV Infusion*<br>• Initially 1 mg (base) as a test dose, administered in 20 mL of 5% dextrose injection over a period of 20 to 30 minutes, with 5 mg to 10 mg incremental increases depending on patient tolerance and severity of the infection, up to a maximum of 0.5 mg/kg to 0.7 mg/kg<br>• Should be infused over a period of 2 to 6 hours |

*Editors' Notes:*

Universal concomitant nephrotoxicity with cyclosporine-A. Requires close dose monitoring. Hydration prior to dosing may help prevent renal toxicity. Renal toxicity is usually reversible.

# Amphotericin B Lipid Complex Injection

| | |
|---|---|
| **Brand Name** | Ambelcet™ |
| **Company** | The Liposome Company, Inc. |
| **Class** | • Antifungal polyene antibiotic obtained from a strain of *Streptomyces nodosus* |
| **Mechanism of Action** | • Binds to sterols in fungus cell membrane, resulting in an inability to function as a selective barrier and a subsequent loss of essential cellular components |
| **Indication** | • Aspergillosis in patients who are refractory to or intolerant of conventional amphotericin B therapy |
| **Contraindication** | • Hypersensitivity to amphotericin B |
| **Warning** | • Anaphylaxis has been reported with amphotericin B-containing products—facilities equipped for cardiopulmonary resuscitation should be available during administration |
| **Special Precautions** | • Pregnancy Category B<br>• It is important to monitor the following patient parameters<br>  • Serum creatinine<br>  • Liver function<br>  • Complete blood count<br>  • Serum magnesium and potassium |
| **Adverse Reactions** | • Infusion-related illness (fever, chills, nausea, vomiting) |
| **Drug Interactions** | • Antineoplastic agents<br>• Corticosteroids and corticotropin<br>• Cyclosporine-A<br>• Digitalis glycosides<br>• Flucytosine<br>• Imidazoles<br>• Leukocyte transfusions<br>• Nephrotoxic medications<br>• Skeletal muscle relaxants<br>• Zidovudine |
| **Formulation** | • Injection |
| **Dosage** | • 5 mg/kg/d IV for invasive aspergillosis<br>• 2.0 mg/kg/d to 2.5 mg/kg/d IV for candidiasis |

# Miconazole Vaginal Cream 2%

| | |
|---|---|
| **Brand Name** | Monistat-Derm® |
| **Company** | Ortho-McNeil Pharmaceutical |
| **Class** | • Synthetic antifungal agent with activity against common dermatophytes including *Trichophyton rubrum, Trichophyton mentagrophytes,* and *Epidermophyton floccosum,* yeast-like fungi such as *Candida albicans,* and *Malassezia furfur,* the organism responsible for tinea versicolor |
| **Mechanism of Action** | • Inhibits growth of dermatophytes and yeast-like fungi |
| **Indications** | • Treatment of tinea pedis, tinea cruris, and tinea corporis caused by susceptible organisms<br>• Treatment of cutaneous candidiasis<br>• Treatment of tinea versicolor |
| **Contraindication** | • None noted |
| **Warning** | • None noted |
| **Special Precautions** | • Treatment should be discontinued if there are signs of sensitivity or chemical irritation<br>• Cream is for external use only |
| **Adverse Reactions** | • Irritation<br>• Burning<br>• Maceration<br>• Allergic contact dermatitis |
| **Drug Interactions** | • None reported |
| **Formulation** | • Cream containing miconazole nitrate at 2% strength, supplied in 15 g, 1 oz, and 3 oz tubes |
| **Dosage** | *Tinea Pedis, Tinea Cruris, Tinea Corporis, and Cutaneous Candidiasis*<br>• Enough to cover affected areas twice daily (morning and evening)<br><br>*Tinea Versicolor*<br>• Enough to cover affected areas once daily |

# Ketoconazole

| | |
|---|---|
| **Brand Name** | Nizoral® |
| **Company** | Janssen Pharmaceutica |
| **Class** | • Synthetic broad-spectrum antifungal agent with clinical activity against *Blastomyces dermatitidis, Candida* species, *Coccidioides immitis, Histoplasma capsulatum, Paracoccidioides brasiliensis, Phialophora* species, *Trichophyton* species, *Epidermophyton* species, and *Microsporum* species |
| **Mechanism of Action** | • Impairs the synthesis of ergosterol, which is a vital component of fungus cell membranes |
| **Indications** | • Treatment of the following systemic fungal infections:<br>• Candidiasis • Chronic mucocutaneous candidiasis<br>• Oral thrush • Candiduria<br>• Blastomycosis • Coccidioidomycosis<br>• Histoplasmosis • Chromomycosis<br>• Paracoccidioidomycosis |
| **Contraindications** | • Hypersensitivity to ketoconazole<br>• Concurrent use of terfenadine or astemizole |
| **Warnings** | • Hepatotoxicity, primarily of the hepatocellular type, has been reported<br>• Anaphylaxis may occur after the first dose<br>• Deaths within 2 weeks of treatment initiation have been reported in patients with prostate cancer; the role of ketoconazole in these deaths has not been ascertained, but it is known that ketoconazole can suppress adrenal corticosteroid secretion |
| **Special Precautions** | • Ketoconazole has been shown to lower serum testosterone<br>• Drug-induced achlorhydria can cause reduction in absorption of ketoconazole<br>• Pregnancy Category C |
| **Adverse Reactions** | • Nausea/vomiting • Abdominal pain • Pruritus |
| **Drug Interactions** | • May enhance anticoagulant effects of coumarin-like drugs<br>• Rifampin • INH • Cyclosporine<br>• Phenytoin • Hypoglycemic agents • Terfenadine<br>• Astemizole |
| **Formulations** | • Tablets containing 200 mg of ketoconazole, supplied in bottles of 100 tablets and in blister packs of 10 X 10 tablets<br>• Also available in cream and shampoo formulations |
| **Dosage** | *Adults*<br>• 200 mg in a single daily administration<br>• If there is insufficient response, dose can be raised to 400 mg/d<br><br>*Children*<br>• 3.3 mg/kg to 6.6 mg/kg in a single daily dose |

*Editors' Notes:*

Ketoconazole has been used in cardiac and renal transplant recipients to lower cyclosporine doses. The long-term safety of this approach has not been established.

# Chapter 3
# Cardiovascular Agents

## Cardiovascular Agents Overview

## Calcium Channel Blockers

- Diltiazem
- Nifedipine
- Isradipine
- Verapamil
- Amlodipine
- Amlodipine and benazepril

## Alpha-Adrenergic Receptor Blockers

- Terazosin
- Clonidine
- Doxazosin
- Labetalol

## Beta-Blockers

- Metoprolol
- Atenolol

## ACE Inhibitors

- Lisinopril
- Enalapril
- Captopril

## Cholesterol-Lowering Agents

- Lovastatin
- Pravastatin
- Fluvastatin
- Simvastatin

# Cardiovascular Agents Overview

| Agent | Dosage |
|---|---|
| **Calcium Channel Blockers** | • Dosage should be individualized by titration<br>*Diltiazem*<br>• 180 mg/d to 240 mg/d<br>*Nifedipine*<br>• 30 mg/d or 60 mg/d<br>*Isradipine*<br>• 2.5 mg BID alone or in combination with a thiazide diuretic<br>*Verapamil*<br>• 180 mg/d with upward titrations if adequate response is not obtained<br>*Amlodipine*<br>• 5 mg/d with a maximum dose of 10 mg/d<br>*Amlodipine and benazepril hydrochloride*<br>• 2.5 mg to 5 mg of amlodipine and 10 mg to 20 mg of benazepril once daily |
| **Alpha-Adrenergic Receptor Blockers** | • Dosage must be individualized<br>*Terazosin*<br>• Initial dosage is 1 mg at bedtime<br>• Maintenance range is usually 1 mg/d to 5 mg/d<br>*Clonidine*<br>• Initial dosage is 0.1 mg twice a day<br>• Maintenance dose is reached with 0.1 mg/d increments until patient reaches the appropriate maintenance range of 0.2 mg/d to 0.6 mg/d given in divided doses<br>*Doxazosin*<br>• Initial dosage is 1 mg given once daily<br>• Depending on standing blood pressure, dose may be increased to 2 mg and then if necessary to 4 mg, 8 mg, or 16 mg<br>*Labetalol ($\alpha$- and $\beta$-blocker)*<br>• 100 mg twice daily<br>• After 2 or 3 days, dosage may be titrated in increments of 100 mg BID every 2 or 3 days; usual maintenance range is 200 mg to 400 mg twice daily |
| **Beta-Blockers** | • Dosage must be individualized<br>*Metoprolol*<br>• Initial dosage is 100 mg/d in single or divided doses alone or added to diuretic therapy<br>• Dosage can be increased at weekly (or longer intervals) until optimal control is achieved, usually at 100 mg/d to 450 mg/d<br>*Atenolol*<br>• Initial dosage is 50 mg/d given as 1 tablet alone or added to diuretic therapy<br>• If optimal effect is not achieved within 1 to 2 weeks, dosage can be increased to 100 mg/d given as a single tablet |

*Continued ...*

# Cardiovascular Agents Overview

| Agent | Dosage |
|---|---|
| **ACE Inhibitors** | • Dosage should be individualized<br><br>*Lisinopril*<br>• Initial dosage is 10 mg/d given once a day<br>• Usual maintenance range is 20 mg/d to 40 mg/d in a single dose<br><br>*Enalapril*<br>• Initial dosage is 5 mg/d given once a day<br>• Usual maintenance range is 10 mg/d to 40 mg/d in a single dose or in 2 divided doses<br><br>*Captopril*<br>• Initial dosage is 25 mg BID or TID<br>• If optimal effect is not achieved within 1 to 2 weeks, dosage can be increased to 50 mg BID or TID |
| **Cholesterol-Lowering Agents** | • Dosage should be individualized<br><br>*Lovastatin*<br>• Initial dosage is 20 mg/d taken once daily with the evening meal<br>• Patients on immunosuppressive therapy should be started on 10 mg/d and should not exceed 20 mg/d<br>• Maximum recommended dose is 80 mg/d<br><br>*Pravastatin*<br>• Starting dose is 10 mg/d or 20 mg/d taken once daily at bedtime<br>• Patients on immunosuppressive therapy should be started on 10 mg/d and should not exceed 20 mg/d<br><br>*Fluvastatin*<br>• Initial dose is 20 mg/d at bedtime<br>• Recommended dosage range is 20 mg/d to 40 mg/d as a single dose<br><br>*Simvastatin*<br>• Starting dosage range is 5 mg/d to 10 mg/d<br>• Maximum dosage is 40 mg/d |

# Calcium Channel Blockers

| Brand Name | Cardizem® CD (diltiazem) | Procardia® XL (nifedipine) | DynaCirc® (isradipine) |
|---|---|---|---|
| **Company** | Marion Merrell Dow Inc. | Pratt Division / Pfizer | Novartis |
| **Mechanism of Action** | • Modulate influx of ionic calcium across the cell membrane of arterial smooth muscle as well as in conductile and contractile myocardial cells | | |
| **Indication** | • Management of essential hypertension | | |
| **Contraindications** | • Hypersensitivity to diltiazem<br>• Hypotension<br>• Sick sinus syndrome<br>• Second- or third-degree AV block<br>• Acute myocardial infarction and pulmonary congestion | • Hypersensitivity to nifedipine | • Hypersensitivity to isradipine |
| **Adverse Reactions** | • Headache<br>• Bradycardia<br>• Edema<br>• Dizziness<br>• ECG abnormalities<br>• AV block first degree<br>• Asthenia | • Edema<br>• Headache<br>• Fatigue<br>• Dizziness<br>• Constipation<br>• Nausea | • Headache<br>• Dizziness<br>• Edema<br>• Palpitations<br>• Fatigue<br>• Flushing |
| **Drug Interactions** | • Other antihypertensive agents (vasodilators, ACE inhibitors, diuretics, and beta-blockers)<br>• Digoxin<br>• Disopyramide<br>• Flecainide<br>• Quinidine<br>• Cimetidine<br>• Lithium<br>• Carbamazepine<br>• Rifampin<br>• Phenobarbital<br>• Cyclosporine<br>• Theophylline<br>• Inhalation anesthetics<br>• Neuromuscular blocking agents | | |

*Continued ...*

Immuno-suppression | Antimicrobials | Cardiovascular Agents | Antiosteo-porosis Agents | Antiplatelets | Diabetes Agents | Ulcer Treatment | Diuretics | Other Agents

# Calcium Channel Blockers

| Brand Name | Calan® SR (verapamil) | Norvasc® (amlodipine) | Lotrel™ (amlodipine and benazepril hydrochloride) |
|---|---|---|---|
| Company | G.D. Searle & Co. | Pfizer Inc. | Novartis |
| Mechanism of Action | • Modulate influx of ionic calcium across the cell membrane of arterial smooth muscle as well as in conductile and contractile myocardial cells | | |
| Indication | • Management of essential hypertension | | |
| Contraindications | • Hypersensitivity to verapamil<br>• Severe left ventricular dysfunction<br>• Hypotension<br>• Sick sinus syndrome<br>• Second- or third-degree AV block<br>• Atrial flutter or atrial fibrillation and an accessory bypass tract | • Hypersensitivity to amlodipine | • Hypersensitivity to amlodipine, benazepril, or any other ACE inhibitor |
| Adverse Reactions | • Constipation<br>• Dizziness<br>• Nausea<br>• Hypotension<br>• Headache<br>• Edema<br>• CHF/pulmonary edema<br>• Fatigue<br>• Dyspnea<br>• Bradycardia<br>• AV block<br>• Rash<br>• Flushing<br>• Elevated hepatic enzymes | • Edema<br>• Dizziness<br>• Flushing<br>• Palpitations | • Cough<br>• Headache<br>• Dizziness<br>• Edema |
| Drug Interactions | • Other antihypertensive agents (vasodilators, ACE inhibitors, diuretics, and beta-blockers)<br>• Digoxin<br>• Disopyramide<br>• Flecainide<br>• Quinidine<br>• Cimetidine<br>• Lithium<br>• Carbamazepine<br>• Rifampin<br>• Phenobarbital<br>• Cyclosporine<br>• Theophylline<br>• Inhalation anesthetics<br>• Neuromuscular blocking agents | • None known | • Diuretics<br>• Potassium supplements or potassium-sparing diuretics<br>• Lithium |

*Continued ...*

# Calcium Channel Blockers

| Brand Name | Cardizem® CD (diltiazem) | Procardia® XL (nifedipine) | DynaCirc® (isradipine) |
|---|---|---|---|
| **Dosage** | • Dose should be individualized by titration<br>• 180 mg/d to 240 mg/d | • Dose should be individualized by titration<br>• 30 mg/d or 60 mg/d | • Dose should be individualized<br>• 2.5 mg BID alone or in combination with a thiazide diuretic |

*Continued ...*

# Calcium Channel Blockers

| Brand Name | Calan® SR (verapamil) | Norvasc® (amlopidine) | Lotrel™ (amlopidine and benazepril hydrochloride) |
|---|---|---|---|
| Dosage | • Dose should be individualized by titration<br>• 180 mg/d with upward titrations if adequate response is not obtained | • Dose should be individualized<br>• 5 mg/d with a maximum dose of 10 mg/d | • Dose should be individualized by titration<br>• 2.5 mg to 5 mg amlodipine and 10 mg to 20 mg of benazepril once daily |

*Editors' Notes:*

Calcium channel blockers are considered the drug of first choice for the treatment of posttransplant hypertension since they increase renal blood flow. Nifedipine and isradipine show little interaction with cyclosporine-A. Diltiazem and verapamil elevate cyclosporine-A levels.

# Alpha-Adrenergic Receptor Blockers

| **Brand Name** | **Hytrin®**<br>**(terazosin)** | **Catapres®**<br>**(clonidine)** | **Cardura®**<br>**(doxazosin)** | **Normodyne®**<br>**(labetalol)**<br>**(α- and β-blocker)** |
|---|---|---|---|---|
| **Company** | Abbott Laboratories | Boehringer Ingelheim Pharmaceuticals, Inc. | Roerig Division/Pfizer | Schering Corporation |
| **Mechanism of Action** | • Block alpha-adrenoreceptors in the brain stem, resulting in reduced sympathetic outflow from the CNS and a decrease in peripheral vascular resistance | | | |
| **Indication** | • Management of hypertension | | | |
| **Contraindications** | • None reported | • None reported | • Known sensitivity to quinazolines | • Bronchial asthma<br>• Overt cardiac failure<br>• AV block (>1st degree)<br>• Severe bradycardia |
| **Special Consideration** | • Alpha-adrenergic agents can cause marked hypotension after the first dose, especially in the upright position, with syncope and other postural symptoms | | | |
| **Adverse Reactions** | • Dizziness<br>• Headache<br>• Asthenia<br>• Nasal congestion<br>• Peripheral edema<br>• Somnolence<br>• Nausea<br>• Palpitations<br>• Pain-extremities<br>• Paresthesia<br>• Dyspnea<br>• Sinusitis<br>• Back pain<br>• Nervousness<br>• Tachycardia<br>• Blurred vision<br>• Postural hypotension<br>• Impotence | • Dry mouth<br>• Drowsiness<br>• Dizziness<br>• Constipation<br>• Sedation | • Dizziness<br>• Nausea<br>• Fatigue<br>• Dyspepsia<br>• Nasal stuffiness<br>• Headache<br>• Ejaculation failure<br>• Dyspnea<br>• Vertigo<br>• Asthenia<br>• Taste distortion<br>• Sexual dysfunction<br>• Edema<br>• Postural hypotension<br>• Rash<br>• Vision abnormality | • Dizziness<br>• Fatigue<br>• Nausea<br>• Vomiting<br>• Dyspepsia<br>• Paresthesia<br>• Nasal stuffiness<br>• Ejaculation failure<br>• Impotence<br>• Edema |
| **Drug Interactions** | • None reported | • Anti-depressants<br>• CNS depressants (alcohol, barbiturates, and other sedatives) | • None reported | • Antidepressants<br>• Beta-blockers<br>• Cimetidine<br>• Nitroglycerin |

*Continued ...*

# Alpha-Adrenergic Receptor Blockers

| Brand Name | Hytrin® (terazosin) | Catapres® (clonidine) | Cardura® (doxazosin) | Normodyne® (labetalol) (α- and β-blocker) |
|---|---|---|---|---|
| **Dosage** | • Dosage must be individualized<br>• Initial dosage is 1 mg at bedtime<br>• Maintenance range is usually 1 mg/d to 5 mg/d | • Dosage must be individualized<br>• Initial dosage is 0.1 mg twice a day<br>• Maintenance dose is reached with 0.1 mg/d increments until patient reaches the appropriate maintenance range of 0.2 mg/d to 0.6 mg/d given in divided doses | • Dosage must be individualized<br>• Initial dosage is 1 mg given once daily<br>• Depending on standing blood pressure, dose may be increased to 2 mg and then if necessary to 4 mg, 8 mg, or 16 mg | • 100 mg twice daily<br>• After 2 or 3 days, dosage may be titrated in increments of 100 mg BID every 2 or 3 days; usual maintenance range is 200 mg to 400 mg twice daily |

*Editors' Notes:*

Clonidine is useful in diabetic patients because there is no effect on lipids or on glucose metabolism.

# Beta-Blockers

| Brand Name | Lopressor® (metoprolol) | Tenormin® (atenolol) |
|---|---|---|
| **Company** | Novartis | Zeneca Pharmaceuticals |
| **Mechanism of Action** | Not known, but the following have been suggested:<br>• Competitive antagonism of catecholamines at peripheral adrenergic neuron sites, leading to decreased cardiac output<br>• Suppression of renin activity | |
| **Indication** | • Management of hypertension | |
| **Contraindications** | • Sinus bradycardia<br>• Heart block (>1st degree)<br>• Cardiogenic shock<br>• Overt cardiac failure | |
| **Special Consideration** | • Patients with bronchospastic disease should not receive therapy with beta-blockers | |
| **Adverse Reactions** | • Tiredness<br>• Dizziness<br>• Depression<br>• Diarrhea<br>• Pruritus/rash<br>• Shortness of breath<br>• Bradycardia<br>• Cold extremities<br>• Arterial insufficiency (Raynaud type)<br>• Palpitations<br>• CHF<br>• Peripheral edema<br>• Hypotension<br>• Bronchospasm<br>• Dyspnea<br>• Nausea<br>• Dry mouth<br>• Gastric pain<br>• Constipation<br>• Flatulence<br>• Heartburn | • Dizziness<br>• Nausea<br>• Bradycardia<br>• Fatigue<br>• Postural hypotension<br>• Vertigo<br>• Diarrhea<br>• Light-headedness<br>• Lethargy |
| **Drug Interactions** | • Catecholamine-depleting drugs (reserpine)<br>• Clonidine<br>• Verapamil<br>• Epinephrine (in patients with history of severe anaphylactic reactions to a variety of allergens) | |
| **Dosage** | • Dosage must be individualized<br>• Initial dosage is 100 mg/d in single or divided doses alone or added to diuretic therapy<br>• Dosage can be increased at weekly (or longer intervals) until optimal control is achieved, usually at 100 mg/d to 450 mg/d | • Dosage must be individualized<br>• Initial dosage is 50 mg/d given as 1 tablet alone or added to diuretic therapy<br>• If optimal effect is not achieved within 1 to 2 weeks, dosage can be increased to 100 mg/d given as a single tablet |

*Editors' Notes:*

Beta-blockers are contraindicated in diabetics and in patients with peripheral vascular disease.

# ACE Inhibitors

| **Brand Name** | **Prinivil® (lisinopril)**<br>**Zestril® (lisinopril)** | **Vasotec® (enalapril)** | **Capoten® (captopril)** |
|---|---|---|---|
| **Company** | Merck & Co., Inc.<br>Zeneca Pharmaceuticals | Merck & Co., Inc. | Bristol-Myers Squibb Co. |
| **Mechanism of Action** | • Inhibit angiotensin-converting enzyme (ACE), resulting in decreased plasma angiotensin II which leads to decreased vasopressor activity and decreased aldosterone secretion | | |
| **Indication** | • Treatment of hypertension | | |
| **Contraindications** | • Hypersensitivity to agent<br>• History of angioedema related to previous ACE inhibitor treatment | | |
| **Adverse Reactions** | • Dizziness<br>• Headache<br>• Fatigue<br>• Diarrhea<br>• Upper respiratory symptoms<br>• Cough<br>• Nausea<br>• Hypotension<br>• Rash<br>• Orthostatic effects<br>• Asthenia<br>• Chest pain<br>• Vomiting<br>• Dyspnea<br>• Dyspepsia | • Headache<br>• Dizziness<br>• Fatigue<br>• Diarrhea<br>• Nausea<br>• Rash<br>• Cough<br>• Orthostatic effects<br>• Asthenia | • Rash, often with pruritus, and sometimes fever, arthralgia, and eosinophilia<br>• Dysgeusia<br>• Cough<br>• Proteinuria<br>• Hypotension<br>• Tachycardia<br>• Chest pain<br>• Palpitations<br>• Angioedema |
| **Drug Interactions** | • Diuretics<br>• Indomethacin<br>• Agents increasing serum potassium<br>• Lithium<br>• Agents causing renin release<br>• Agents affecting sympathetic activity | | |
| **Dosage** | • Initial dosage is 10 mg/d given once a day<br>• Dose should be individually adjusted according to blood pressure response<br>• Usual maintenance range is 20 mg/d to 40 mg/d in a single dose | • Initial dosage is 5 mg/d given once a day<br>• Dose should be individually adjusted according to blood pressure response<br>• Usual maintenance range is 10 mg/d to 40 mg/d in a single dose or in 2 divided doses | • Dosage must be individualized and captopril tablets should be taken 1 hour before meals<br>• Initial dosage is 25 mg BID or TID<br>• If optimal effect is not achieved within 1 to 2 weeks, dosage can be increased to 50 mg BID or TID |

*Editors' Notes:*

Enalapril may cause anemia. It has been used successfully in low doses for posttransplant polycythemia. ACE inhibitors may precipitate renal failure in patients with renal transplant artery stenosis. A rapid rise in serum creatinine after initiation of ACE inhibitor therapy may indicate renal transplant artery stenosis.

# Cholesterol-Lowering Agents

| Brand Name | Mevacor® (lovastatin) | Pravachol® (pravastatin) |
|---|---|---|
| Company | Merck & Co., Inc. | Bristol-Myers Squibb Co. |
| Mechanism of Action | • Inhibit HMG-CoA reductase, preventing the conversion of HMG-CoA to mevalonate, an early step in cholesterol biosynthesis<br>• Depletion of cellular cholesterol stimulates the production of cell surface receptors that recognize LDL, leading to increased catabolism of LDL cholesterol | |
| Indication | • Adjunct to diet for the reduction of elevated total and LDL cholesterol levels in patients with primary hypercholesterolemia (Types IIa and IIb) when the response to a diet restricted in saturated fat and cholesterol and to other nonpharmacologic measures has been inadequate | |
| Contraindications | • Hypersensitivity to any component of these medications<br>• Active liver disease<br>• Pregnancy and lactation (Pregnancy Category X) | |
| Adverse Reactions | • Headache<br>• Flatus<br>• Abdominal pain and cramps<br>• Diarrhea<br>• Rash/Pruritus<br>• Constipation<br>• Nausea<br>• Dyspepsia<br>• Myalgia<br>• Dizziness<br>• Heartburn<br>• Blurred vision<br>• Muscle cramps | • Localized pain<br>• Nausea/vomiting<br>• Common cold<br>• Diarrhea<br>• Headache<br>• Abdominal pain<br>• Cardiac chest pain<br>• Rash<br>• Constipation<br>• Rhinitis<br>• Fatigue<br>• Chest pain<br>• Flatulence<br>• Dizziness<br>• Heartburn<br>• Myalgia<br>• Cough<br>• Influenza<br>• Urinary abnormality |
| Drug Interactions | • Cyclosporine<br>• Gemfibrozil<br>• Niacin<br>• Erythromycin<br>• Cholestyramine/Colestipol<br>• Warfarin<br>• Cimetidine<br>• Digoxin | |
| Dosage | • Dosage should be individualized<br>• Initial dosage is 20 mg/d taken once daily with the evening meal<br>• Patients on immunosuppressive therapy should be started on 10 mg/d and should not exceed 20 mg/d<br>• Maximum recommended dose is 80 mg/d | • Dosage should be individualized<br>• Starting dose is 10 mg/d or 20 mg/d taken once daily at bedtime<br>• Patients on immunosuppressive therapy should be started on 10 mg/d and should not exceed 20 mg/d |

*Continued ...*

# Cholesterol-Lowering Agents

| Brand Name | Lescol® (fluvastatin sodium) | Zocor® (simvastatin) |
|---|---|---|
| **Company** | Novartis | Merck & Co., Inc. |
| **Mechanism of Action** | • Inhibit HMG-CoA reductase, preventing the conversion of HMG-CoA to mevalonate, an early step in cholesterol biosynthesis<br>• Depletion of cellular cholesterol stimulates the production of cell surface receptors that recognize LDL, leading to increased catabolism of LDL cholesterol | |
| **Indication** | • Adjunct to diet for the reduction of elevated total and LDL cholesterol levels in patients with primary hypercholesterolemia (Types IIa and IIb) when the response to a diet restricted in saturated fat and cholesterol and to other nonpharmacologic measures has been inadequate | |
| **Contraindications** | • Hypersensitivity to any component of these medications<br>• Active liver disease<br>• Pregnancy and lactation (Pregnancy Category X) | |
| **Adverse Reactions** | Adverse events with a higher incidence in fluvastatin-treated patients than placebo patients<br>• Arthropathy<br>• Exercise-related muscle pain<br>• Sinusitis<br>• Bronchitis<br>• Dyspepsia<br>• Diarrhea<br>• Abdominal pain<br>• Nausea<br>• Insomnia<br>• Fatigue | • Abdominal pain<br>• Asthenia<br>• Constipation<br>• Diarrhea<br>• Dyspepsia<br>• Flatulence<br>• Nausea<br>• Headache<br>• Upper respiratory tract infection |
| **Drug Interactions** | • Gemfibrozil<br>• Niacin<br>• Erythromycin<br>• Cholestyramine<br>• Digoxin<br>• Cimetidine/ranitidine/omeprazole<br>• Rifampicin<br>• Warfarin | • Itraconazole<br>• Gemfibrozil<br>• Niacin<br>• Erythromycin<br>• Propranolol<br>• Digoxin<br>• Warfarin |
| **Dosage** | • Initial dosage is 20 mg/d at bedtime<br>• Recommended dosage range is 20 mg/d to 40 mg/d as a single dose | • Dosage should be individualized according to baseline LDL-C levels<br>• Starting dosage range is 5 mg/d to 10 mg/d<br>• Maximum dosage is 40 mg/d |

*Editors' Notes:*

Cyclosporine prolongs the half-life of statin drugs. Therefore, in transplant recipients, the preferred dose of these cholesterol-lowering agents is half of the recommended dose. Some of these agents have been reported to cause rhabdomyolysis when given to patients receiving cyclosporine-A.

# Chapter 4
# Antiosteoporosis Agents

## Antiosteoporosis Agents Overview

- Alendronate Sodium
- Etidronate Disodium
- Calcitonin-salmon

# Antiosteoporosis Agents Overview

| Agent | Dosage |
|---|---|
| **Alendronate sodium** | *Postmenopausal Osteoporosis*<br>• 10 mg/d with a full glass of ***plain*** water<br><br>*Paget's Disease*<br>• 40 mg/d for 6 months |
| **Etidronate disodium** | *Paget's Disease*<br>• 5 mg/kg/d to 10 mg/kg/d for a period not to exceed 6 months or 11 mg/kg/d to 20 mg/kg/d for no longer than 3 months<br><br>*Heterotopic Ossification*<br>• Total hip replacement: 20 mg/kg/d for 1 month before surgery and 3 months after surgery<br>• Spinal cord injury: 20 mg/kg/d for 2 weeks followed by 10 mg/kg/d for 10 weeks |
| **Calcitonin-salmon** | • 200 IU/d intranasally, alternating nostrils daily |

*Editors' Notes:*

Although these agents are not indicated for the prevention of steroid-induced bone loss, they are useful for the many patients who have significant osteoporosis prior to transplantation. Rapid bone loss occurs after transplantation, placing these patients at increased risk for fractures. Because of improving long-term survival, attention to metabolic bone disease should occur early in the posttransplant course so that the risk of complications might be lessened.

# Alendronate Sodium

| | |
|---|---|
| **Brand Name** | Fosamax® |
| **Company** | Merck & Co., Inc. |
| **Class** | • Hormone-free antiosteoporosis agent |
| **Mechanism of Action** | • Reduces activity of cells that cause bone loss, thereby reducing the rate of bone loss and increasing bone density |
| **Indications** | • Postmenopausal osteoporosis<br>• Paget's disease having alkaline phosphatase at least two times the upper limit of normal, or in patients who are symptomatic or at risk for further complications |
| **Contraindications** | • Hypersensitivity to any component of this product<br>• Hypocalcemia |
| **Special Precautions** | • Not recommended for patients with renal insufficiencies<br>• Should be used with caution in patients with gastrointestinal problems<br>• Hypocalcemia should be corrected before initiating therapy<br>• Pregnancy Category C |
| **Adverse Reactions** | • Abdominal pain<br>• Nausea<br>• Dyspepsia<br>• Constipation<br>• Diarrhea<br>• Flatulence<br>• Acid regurgitation<br>• Esophageal ulcer<br>• Vomiting<br>• Dysphagia<br>• Abdominal distention<br>• Gastritis<br>• Taste perversion<br>• Headache<br>• Dizziness<br>• Muscle cramp<br>• Musculoskeletal pain |
| **Drug Interactions** | • Estrogen<br>• Calcium supplements/antacids<br>• NSAIDs |
| **Formulation** | • Tablets |
| **Dosage** | *Postmenopausal Osteoporosis*<br>• 10 mg/d with a full glass of ***plain*** water<br><br>*Paget's Disease*<br>• 40 mg/d for 6 months |

*Editors' Notes:*

Major side effects include GI symptoms. Renal insufficiency may preclude use.

# Etidronate Disodium

| | |
|---|---|
| **Brand Name** | Didronel® |
| **Company** | Procter & Gamble Pharmaceuticals, Inc. |
| **Class** | • Bone metabolism regulator |
| **Mechanism of Action** | • Inhibits formation, growth, and dissolution of hydroxyapatite crystals and their amorphous precursors by chemisorption to calcium phosphate surfaces |
| **Indications** | • Symptomatic Paget's disease of bone<br>• Heterotopic ossification |
| **Contraindications** | • Known hypersensitivity to etidronate disodium<br>• Clinically overt osteomalacia |
| **Warning** | • In Paget's patients, onset of effect may be slow |
| **Special Precautions** | • Patients should maintain adequate intake of calcium and vitamin D<br>• Patients with enterocolitis may experience diarrhea<br>• Etidronate is not metabolized and is excreted intact via the kidney<br>• Pregnancy Category C |
| **Adverse Reactions** | • Gastrointestinal complaints<br>• Increased pain at previously asymptomatic pagetic sites<br>• Alopecia<br>• Arthropathies<br>• Bone fracture<br>• Esophagitis/glossitis<br>• Hypersensitivity reactions |
| **Drug Interactions** | • None reported |
| **Formulation** | • 200 mg tablets |
| **Dosage** | *Paget's Disease*<br>• 5 mg/kg/d to 10 mg/kg/d for a period not to exceed 6 months or 11 mg/kg/d to 20 mg/kg/d for no longer than 3 months<br><br>*Heterotopic Ossification*<br>• Total hip replacement: 20 mg/kg/d for 1 month before surgery and 3 months after surgery<br>• Spinal cord injury: 20 mg/kg/d for 2 weeks followed by 10 mg/kg/d for 10 weeks |

*Editors' Notes:*

Usually given in cycles—2 weeks of etidronate followed by 10 weeks of calcium and vitamin D.

# Calcitonin-Salmon

| | |
|---|---|
| **Brand Name** | Miacalcin® |
| **Company** | Novartis |
| **Class** | • Synthetic polypeptide hormone with the same linear sequence of amino acids as calcitonin of salmon origin |
| **Mechanism of Action** | • Causes transient inhibition of the bone resorptive process possibly through inhibition of osteoclast function with loss of the ruffled osteoclast border responsible for resorption of bone |
| **Indication** | • Postmenopausal osteoporosis |
| **Contraindication** | • Clinical allergy to calcitonin-salmon |
| **Warning** | • Possibility of systemic allergic reaction exists because calcitonin-salmon is a polypeptide |
| **Special Precautions** | • Periodic nasal examinations are recommended<br>• Pregnancy Category C |
| **Adverse Reactions** | • Rhinitis and other nasal symptoms<br>• Back pain<br>• Arthralgia<br>• Epistaxis<br>• Headache |
| **Drug Interactions** | • No drug interaction studies have been conducted<br>• No drug interactions have been observed |
| **Formulation** | • Metered dose solution in 2-mL fill glass bottles with a dose strength of 200 IU per activation (0.09 mL/puff) |
| **Dosage** | • 200 IU/d intranasally, alternating nostrils daily |

*Editors' Notes:*

New agent with little experience in transplant recipients.

# Chapter 5
# Antiplatelets

## Antiplatelets Overview

- Aspirin

# Antiplatelets Overview

| Agent | Dosage |
|---|---|
| **Aspirin** | *Transient Ischemic Attack*<br>• 1300 mg/d given in divided doses of 650 mg 2 times a day or 325 mg 4 times a day<br><br>*Myocardial Infarction*<br>• 325 mg/d |

# Aspirin

| | |
|---|---|
| **Names of Commonly Used Brands** | • Anacin®<br>• Ascriptin®<br>• Bayer® Aspirin<br>• Bufferin®<br>• Easprin®<br>• Ecotrin®<br>• Norwich® Aspirin |
| **Mechanism of Action** | • Inhibits the enzyme prostaglandin cyclooxygenase in platelets, which prevents the formation of the aggregating agent thromboxane $A_2$<br>• May also inhibit formation of prostacyclin, a platelet aggregation inhibitor |
| **Indication** | • Antiplatelet prophylaxis to reduce risk of recurrent transient ischemic attacks (TIA) and myocardial infarction (MI) |
| **Contraindication** | • Hypersensitivity to aspirin |
| **Adverse Reactions** | • Stomach pain<br>• Heartburn<br>• Nausea/vomiting<br>• Increased rates of gross gastrointestinal bleeding<br>• Small increases in systolic blood pressure<br>• Slight increases in BUN and uric acid levels |
| **Drug Interactions** | • Acetaminophen<br>• Acidifiers, urinary (ammonium chloride, ascorbic acid, potassium or sodium phosphates)<br>• Adrenocorticoids, glucocorticoids, and corticotropin<br>• NSAIDs<br>• Alkalizers, urinary (carbonic anhydrase inhibitors, citrates, sodium bicarbonate, antacids)<br>• Anticoagulants<br>• Heparin or thrombolytic agents<br>• Hydantoin<br>• Antidiabetic agents<br>• Cefamandole, cefoperazone, cefotetan, moxalactam, plicamycin, valproic acid<br>• Furosemide<br>• Laxatives, cellulose-containing<br>• Methotrexate<br>• Nifedipine, verapamil<br>• Vancomycin<br>• Platelet aggregation inhibitors<br>• Probenecid, sulfinpyrazone<br>• Salicylic acid<br>• Zidovudine |
| **Dosage** | *TIA*<br>• 1300 mg/d given in divided doses of 650 mg 2 times a day or 325 mg 4 times a day<br><br>*MI*<br>• 325 mg/d |

# Chapter 6
# Diabetes Agents

## Diabetes Agents Overview

- Insulin
- Glyburide
- Glipizide
- Metformin

# Diabetes Agents Overview

| Agent | Dosage |
|---|---|
| **Insulin** | *Insulin, Human Isophane Suspension*<br>• Variable regimens<br><br>*Insulin, Human NPH*<br>• Variable regimens<br><br>*Insulin, Human Regular*<br>• Variable regimens<br><br>*Insulin, Human Regular and Human NPH Mixture*<br>• Variable regimens<br><br>*Insulin, Human, Zinc Suspension*<br>• Variable regimens<br><br>*Insulin, NPH*<br>• Variable regimens<br><br>*Insulin, Regular*<br>• Variable regimens<br><br>*Insulin, Regular and NPH Mixture*<br>• Variable regimens<br><br>*Insulin, Zinc Crystals*<br>• Variable regimens<br><br>*Insulin, Zinc Suspension*<br>• Variable regimens |
| **Glyburide** | *Diaβeta®*<br>• Usual starting dose range is 2.5 mg/d to 5 mg/d administered with breakfast or the first main meal<br>• Usual maintenance range is 1.25 mg/d to 20 mg/d given as a single dose or in divided doses<br>• Increments should be no greater than 2.5 mg at weekly intervals<br><br>*Micronase®*<br>• Usual starting dose range is 2.5 mg/d to 5 mg/d administered with breakfast or the first main meal<br>• Usual maintenance range is 1.25 mg/d to 20 mg/d given as a single dose or in divided doses<br>• Increments should be no greater than 2.5 mg at weekly intervals<br><br>*Glynase®*<br>• Patients should be retitrated when transferred from other oral hypoglycemic agents<br>• Usual starting dose range is 1.5 mg/d to 3 mg/d administered with breakfast or the first main meal<br>• Usual maintenance range is 0.75 mg/d to 12 mg/d given as a single dose or in divided doses<br>• Increments should be no greater than 1.5 mg at weekly intervals |

*Continued ...*

# Diabetes Agents Overview

| | |
|---|---|
| **Glipizide** | *Glucotrol®*<br>• Recommended initial dose is 5 mg/d given before breakfast<br>• Dosage adjustments should be made in increments of 2.5 mg to 5 mg<br>• Maximum once-daily dose is 15 mg; dosages above 15 mg should be divided, given before meals of adequate caloric content, and should not exceed 40 mg/d |
| **Metformin hydrochloride** | • Recommended starting dosage is 500 mg BID with meals<br>• Dosage should be increased by one 500 mg tablet each week<br>• Individualize dosage based on effectiveness and tolerance, up to a maximum of 2500 mg/d given in divided doses |

# Insulin

| | |
|---|---|
| **Names of Commonly Used Brands** | *Insulin, Human Isophane Suspension*<br>• Novolin® N<br><br>*Insulin, Human NPH*<br>• Humulin® N<br>• Novolin® N PenFill Cartridges<br>• Insulatard® NPH Human<br><br>*Insulin, Human Regular*<br>• Humulin® BR<br>• Novolin® R<br>• Velosulin® Human<br>• Humulin® R<br>• Novolin® R PenFill Cartridges<br><br>*Insulin, Human Regular and Human NPH Mixture*<br>• Humulin® 50/50<br>• Mixtard® 70/30<br>• Novolin® 70/30 PenFill Cartridges<br>• Humulin® 70/30<br>• Novolin® 70/30<br>• Novolin® 70/30 Prefilled Cartridges<br><br>*Insulin, Human, Zinc Suspension*<br>• Humulin® L<br>• Novolin® L<br>• Humulin® U<br><br>*Insulin, NPH*<br>• NPH Iletin® I<br>• NPH Iletin® II, Pork<br>• NPH Insulin<br>• NPH Iletin® II, Beef<br>• Insulatard® NPH<br>• NPH Purified Pork Isophane Insulin<br><br>*Insulin, Regular*<br>• Iletin® I, Regular<br>• Regular Iletin® II, Pork<br>• Regular Insulin<br>• Regular Purified Pork Insulin<br>• Regular Iletin® II, Beef<br>• Regular Iletin® II (concentrated), Pork<br>• Velosulin®<br><br>*Insulin, Regular and NPH Mixture*<br>• Mixtard® 70/30<br><br>*Insulin, Zinc Crystals*<br>• NPH Iletin® I<br><br>*Insulin, Zinc Suspension*<br>• Iletin® I<br>• Iletin® I, Semilente<br>• Iletin® II<br>• Lente® Iletin® II, Pork<br>• Lente® Purified Pork Insulin<br>• Iletin® I, Lente<br>• Iletin® I, Ultralente<br>• Lente® Iletin® II, Beef<br>• Lente® Insulin<br>• Semilente® Insulin<br>• Ultralente® Insulin |
| **Mechanism of Action** | • Controls the storage and metabolism of carbohydrates, proteins, and fats, influencing cellular growth, enzyme activation and inhibition, and alterations in protein and fat metabolism |

*Continued ...*

# Insulin

| | |
|---|---|
| **Indications** | • Diabetes mellitus, insulin-dependent<br>• Diabetes mellitus, non-insulin-dependent |
| **Contraindication** | • None reported |
| **Adverse Reactions** | • Hypoglycemia (anxious feeling, cold sweats, confusion, cool, pale skin, difficulty in concentration, drowsiness, excessive hunger, headache, nausea, nervousness, rapid pulse, shakiness, unusual tiredness or weakness, vision changes) |
| **Drug Interactions** | • Adrenocorticoids, glucocorticoids<br>• Amphetamines<br>• Baclofen<br>• Contraceptives, oral, estrogen-containing<br>• Corticotropin<br>• Danazol<br>• Dextrothyroxine<br>• Diuretics, thiazide, thiazide-related<br>• Epinephrine<br>• Estrogens<br>• Ethacrynic acid<br>• Furosemide<br>• Glucagon<br>• Molindone<br>• Phenytoin<br>• Thyroid hormones<br>• Triamterene |
| **Dosage** | *Insulin, Human Isophane Suspension*<br>• Variable regimens<br><br>*Insulin, Human NPH*<br>• Variable regimens<br><br>*Insulin, Human Regular*<br>• Variable regimens<br><br>*Insulin, Human Regular and Human NPH Mixture*<br>• Variable regimens<br><br>*Insulin, Human Zinc Suspension*<br>• Variable regimens<br><br>*Insulin, NPH*<br>• Variable regimens<br><br>*Insulin, Regular*<br>• Variable regimens<br><br>*Insulin, Regular and NPH Mixture*<br>• Variable regimens<br><br>*Insulin, Zinc Crystals*<br>• Variable regimens<br><br>*Insulin, Zinc Suspension*<br>• Variable regimens |

# Glyburide

| | |
|---|---|
| **Brand Name/ Company** | • Diaβeta®/Hoechst Marion Roussel Pharmaceuticals, Inc.<br>• Micronase®/Pharmacia and Upjohn, Inc.<br>• Glynase® PresTab®/Pharmacia and Upjohn, Inc. |
| **Mechanism of Action** | • Decreases blood glucose by stimulating the release of insulin from the pancreas in patients with functioning beta cells in the pancreatic islets |
| **Indication** | • Adjunct to diet to lower blood glucose in patients with non-insulin-dependent diabetes mellitus (Type II) whose hyperglycemia cannot be controlled by diet alone |
| **Contraindications** | • Known hypersensitivity or allergy to agent<br>• Diabetic ketoacidosis, with or without coma<br>• Type I diabetes mellitus, as sole therapy (Micronase, Glynase) |
| **Special Consideration** | • Oral hypoglycemic drugs have been associated with increased cardiac mortality as compared to treatment with diet alone or diet and insulin |
| **Adverse Reactions** | • Hypoglycemia<br>• Cholestatic jaundice and hepatitis (therapy should be discontinued)<br>• Liver function abnormalities<br>• Gastrointestinal disturbances (nausea, epigastric fullness, heartburn)<br>• Dermatologic reactions (pruritus, erythema, urticaria, morbilliform)<br>• Hematologic reactions (leukopenia, agranulocytosis, thrombocytopenia, hemolytic anemia, aplastic anemia, pancytopenia)<br>• Metabolic reactions (hepatic porphyria, disulfiram-like reactions)<br>• Hyponatremia |
| **Drug Interactions** | • NSAIDs<br>• Salicylates<br>• Sulfonamides<br>• Chloramphenicol<br>• Probenecid<br>• Coumarins<br>• MAO inhibitors<br>• Beta-blockers<br>• Thiazides and other diuretics<br>• Corticosteroids<br>• Phenothiazines<br>• Thyroid products<br>• Estrogens<br>• Oral contraceptives<br>• Phenytoin<br>• Nicotinic acid<br>• Sympathomimetics<br>• Calcium channel blockers<br>• Isoniazid<br>• Miconazole |

*Continued ...*

# Glyburide

| | |
|---|---|
| **Dosage** | *Diaβeta*<br>• Usual starting dose range is 2.5 mg/d to 5 mg/d administered with breakfast or the first main meal<br>• Usual maintenance range is 1.25 mg/d to 20 mg/d given as a single dose or in divided doses<br>• Increments should be no greater than 2.5 mg at weekly intervals<br><br>*Micronase*<br>• Usual starting dose range is 2.5 mg/d to 5 mg/d administered with breakfast or the first main meal<br>• Usual maintenance range is 1.25 mg/d to 20 mg/d given as a single dose or in divided doses<br>• Increments should be no greater than 2.5 mg at weekly intervals<br><br>*Glynase*<br>• Patients should be retitrated when transferred from other oral hypoglycemic agents<br>• Usual starting dose range is 1.5 mg/d to 3 mg/d administered with breakfast or the first main meal<br>• Usual maintenance range is 0.75 mg/d to 12 mg/d given as a single dose or in divided doses<br>• Increments should be no greater than 1.5 mg at weekly intervals |

*Editors' Notes:*

Glyburide may be given after pancreas transplantation in patients with impaired glucose tolerance.

# Glipizide

| | |
|---|---|
| **Brand Name** | Glucotrol® |
| **Company** | Pratt Division / Pfizer |
| **Mechanism of Action** | • Stimulation of insulin secretion from beta cells of pancreatic islet tissue in patients with functioning beta cells |
| **Indication** | • Adjunct to diet for the control of hyperglycemia and its associated symptomatology in patients with non-insulin-dependent diabetes mellitus (Type II) whose hyperglycemia cannot be controlled by diet alone |
| **Contraindications** | • Known hypersensitivity or allergy to agent<br>• Diabetic ketoacidosis, with or without coma |
| **Special Precautions** | • Oral hypoglycemic drugs have been associated with increased cardiac mortality as compared to treatment with diet alone or diet and insulin |
| **Adverse Reactions** | • Hypoglycemia<br>• Gastrointestinal disturbances (nausea, diarrhea, constipation, gastralgia)<br>• Dermatologic reactions (erythema, morbilliform or maculopapular eruptions, urticaria, pruritus, and eczema)<br>• Hematologic reactions (leukopenia, agranulocytosis, thrombocytopenia, hemolytic anemia, aplastic anemia, pancytopenia)<br>• Metabolic reactions (hepatic porphyria, disulfiram-like reactions)<br>• Hyponatremia<br>• Elevated liver enzymes |
| **Drug Interactions** | • NSAIDs<br>• Sulfonamides<br>• Probenecid<br>• MAO inhibitors<br>• Thiazides and other diuretics<br>• Phenothiazines<br>• Estrogens<br>• Phenytoin<br>• Sympathomimetic<br>• Isoniazid<br>• Salicylates<br>• Chloramphenicol<br>• Coumarins<br>• Beta-blockers<br>• Corticosteroids<br>• Thyroid products<br>• Oral contraceptives<br>• Nicotinic acid<br>• Calcium channel blockers<br>• Miconazole |
| **Dosage** | • Recommended initial dose is 5 mg/d given before breakfast<br>• Dosage adjustments should be made in increments of 2.5 mg to 5 mg<br>• Maximum once-daily dose is 15 mg; dosages above 15 mg should be divided, given before meals of adequate caloric content, and should not exceed 40 mg/d |

# Metformin Hydrochloride

| | |
|---|---|
| **Brand Name** | Glucophage® |
| **Company** | Bristol-Myers Squibb Company |
| **Mechanism of Action** | • Bypasses pancreas and has direct antihyperglycemic action |
| **Indication** | • First-line therapy for the control of hyperglycemia and its associated symptomatology in patients with non-insulin-dependent diabetes mellitus (Type II) |
| **Contraindications** | • Renal disease or renal dysfunction<br>• Should be withheld in patients undergoing radiologic studies involving parenteral administration of iodinated contrast materials<br>• Known hypersensitivity to metformin hydrochloride<br>• Acute or chronic metabolic acidosis, including diabetic ketoacidosis, with or without coma |
| **Warnings** | • Lactic acidosis is a serious metabolic complication that can occur due to metformin accumulation<br>• Oral antidiabetic agents have been associated with an increased risk of cardiovascular mortality as compared to treatment with diet alone or diet and insulin |
| **Special Precautions** | • Renal function should be monitored to minimize risk of metformin accumulation<br>• If hypoxic states occur, discontinue drug therapy<br>• Therapy should be suspended for surgical procedures<br>• Alcohol is known to potentiate the effect of metformin on lactate metabolism—patients should be warned about the dangers of excessive alcohol intake |
| **Adverse Reactions** | • Lactic acidosis<br>• Gastrointestinal disturbances (nausea, vomiting, bloating, flatulence)<br>• Dermatologic reactions (rash/dermatitis)<br>• Hematologic reactions (asymptomatic subnormal serum vitamin $B_{12}$ levels)<br>• Special senses (slight metallic taste upon initiation of therapy) |
| **Drug Interactions** | • Furosemide<br>• Nifedipine<br>• Cationic drugs<br>• Drugs that tend to produce hyperglycemia (thiazide and other diuretics, corticosteroids, phenothiazines, thyroid products, estrogens, oral contraceptives, phenytoin, nicotinic acid, sympathomimetics, calcium channel blockers, isoniazid) |
| **Dosage** | • Recommended starting dosage is 500 mg BID with meals<br>• Dosage should be increased by one 500 mg tablet each week<br>• Individualize dosage based on effectiveness and tolerance, up to a maximum of 2550 mg/d given in divided doses |

*Editors' Notes:*

The major concern is the development of lactic acidosis, which can be fatal. There is little information in the transplant literature regarding metformin.

# Chapter 7
# Ulcer Prophylaxis and Treatment

## Ulcer Prophylaxis and Treatment Overview

## Magnesium/Aluminum Hydroxide Suspension, Aluminum Hydroxide Suspension, Calcium Carbonate

## Histamine $H_2$-Receptor Antagonists

- Famotidine
- Ranitidine
- Cimetidine

## Omeprazole

## Sucralfate

## Misoprostol

# Ulcer Prophylaxis and Treatment Overview

| Agent | Dosage | |
|---|---|---|
| **Magnesium/ Aluminum Hydroxide Suspension** | *Maalox®*<br>• 1 or 2 teaspoons, 4 times a day, taken 20 minutes to 1 hour after meals and at bedtime | |
| **Aluminum Hydroxide Suspension** | *ALternaGEL™*<br>• 1 to 2 teaspoons, as needed, between meals, and at bedtime<br>• May be followed by a sip of water | |
| | *Amphojel®*<br>• 2 teaspoons, followed by a sip of water, 5 to 6 times a day between meals and bedtime | |
| **Calcium Carbonate** | *Tums E-X®*<br>• 1 or 2 tablets as symptoms occur<br>• Patients should take no more than 10 tablets in a 24-hour period | |
| **Histamine $H_2$-Receptor Antagonists** | *Famotidine* | |
| | Duodenal—Acute | • 40 mg once a day at bedtime for up to 6 to 8 weeks |
| | Duodenal—Maintenance | • 20 mg once a day at bedtime |
| | Benign Gastric—Acute | • 40 mg once a day at bedtime |
| | *Ranitidine* | |
| | Duodenal—Acute | • 150 mg or 10 mL twice a day<br>—or—<br>300 mg or 20 mL once a day at bedtime |
| | Duodenal—Maintenance | • 150 mg or 10 mL at bedtime |
| | Benign Gastric | • 150 mg or 10 mL twice a day |
| | *Cimetidine* | |
| | Duodenal—Acute | • 800 mg once daily at bedtime for up to 6 to 8 weeks |
| | Duodenal—Maintenance | • 400 mg at bedtime |
| | Benign Gastric | • 800 mg once daily at bedtime for up to 6 weeks |
| **Omeprazole** | • 20 mg once daily for up to 8 weeks | |
| **Sucralfate** | *Acute Therapy*<br>• 1 g, 4 times a day on an empty stomach for up to 8 weeks | |
| **Misoprostol** | • 200 µg 4 times a day with food for the duration of NSAID therapy | |

# Magnesium/Aluminum Hydroxide Suspension, Aluminum Hydroxide Suspension, Calcium Carbonate

| | | | |
|---|---|---|---|
| **Names of Commonly Used Brands** | *Magnesium/Aluminum*<br>• Maalox®<br>• Maalox® TC | *Aluminum*<br>• ALternaGEL™<br>• Amphojel® | *Calcium*<br>• Tums E-X® Tablets |
| **Mechanism of Action** | • React chemically to neutralize or buffer existing quantities of stomach acid, resulting in an increased pH value of stomach content<br>• Decrease acidity within lumen of the esophagus, causing an increase in intraesophageal pH and a decrease in pepsin activity | | |
| **Indication** | • Symptomatic relief of hyperacidity associated with peptic acid and other gastrointestinal conditions requiring high degree of neutralization | | |
| **Contraindications/ Medical Problems** | • Alzheimer's disease<br>• Appendicitis<br>• Undiagnosed gastrointestinal/ rectal bleeding<br>• Colitis<br>• Colostomy, diverticulitis, or ileostomy<br>• Constipation<br>• Gastric outlet obstruction<br>• Diarrhea<br>• Intestinal obstruction<br>• Hemorrhoids<br>• Renal function impairment<br>• Sensitivity to magnesium or aluminum | • Alzheimer's disease<br>• Appendicitis<br>• Undiagnosed gastrointestinal/ rectal bleeding<br>• Gastric outlet obstruction<br>• Diarrhea<br>• Intestinal obstruction<br>• Hemorrhoids<br>• Renal function impairment<br>• Sensitivity to aluminum | • Hypercalcemia<br>• Appendicitis<br>• Undiagnosed gastrointestinal/rectal bleeding<br>• Constipation<br>• Hypoparathyroidism<br>• Intestinal obstruction<br>• Hemorrhoids<br>• Renal function impairment<br>• Sarcoidosis<br>• Sensitivity to calcium<br>• Diarrhea |
| **Adverse Reactions** | • Hypermagnesemia<br>• Neurotoxicity<br>• Fecal impaction<br>• Hypercalcemia<br>• Osteomalacia and osteoporosis due to phosphate depletion<br>• Phosphorous depletion syndrome | • Neurotoxicity<br>• Fecal impaction<br>• Hypercalcemia<br>• Osteomalacia and osteoporosis due to phosphate depletion<br>• Phosphorous depletion syndrome | • Fecal impaction<br>• Metabolic alkalosis<br>• Hypercalcemia<br>• Renal calculi<br>• Osteomalacia |

*Continued ...*

# Magnesium/Aluminum Hydroxide Suspension, Aluminum Hydroxide Suspension, Calcium Carbonate

| | | | |
|---|---|---|---|
| **Names of Commonly Used Brands** | *Magnesium/Aluminum*<br>• Maalox®<br>• Maalox® TC | *Aluminum*<br>• ALternaGEL™<br>• Amphojel® | *Calcium*<br>• Tums E-X® Tablets |
| **Drug Interactions** | • Urinary acidifiers<br>• Amphetamines or quinidine<br>• Anticholinergics<br>• Chenodiol<br>• Quinolones<br>• Citrates<br>• Digitalis glycosides<br>• Enteric-coated agents<br>• Folic acid<br>• Histamine $H_2$-receptor antagonists<br>• Oral iron preparations<br>• Oral isoniazid<br>• Ketoconazole<br>• Mecamylamine<br>• Methenamine<br>• Misoprostol<br>• Pancrelipase<br>• Penicillamine<br>• Phenothiazines<br>• Phenytoin<br>• Oral phosphates<br>• Salicylates<br>• Sodium fluoride<br>• SPSR<br>• Sucralfate<br>• Tetracyclines<br>• Vitamin D | • Urinary acidifiers<br>• Amphetamines or quinidine<br>• Anticholinergics<br>• Chenodiol<br>• Quinolones<br>• Citrates<br>• Digitalis glycosides<br>• Enteric-coated agents<br>• Folic acid<br>• Histamine $H_2$-receptor antagonists<br>• Oral iron preparations<br>• Oral isoniazid<br>• Ketoconazole<br>• Mecamylamine<br>• Methenamine<br>• Penicillamine<br>• Phenothiazines<br>• Phenytoin<br>• Oral phosphates<br>• Salicylates<br>• Sodium fluoride<br>• Sucralfate<br>• Tetracyclines | • Urinary acidifiers<br>• Amphetamines or quinidine<br>• Anticholinergics<br>• Calcitonin<br>• Cellulose sodium phosphate<br>• Quinolones<br>• Citrates<br>• Diuretics<br>• Enteric-coated agents<br>• Histamine $H_2$-receptor antagonists<br>• Oral iron preparations<br>• Ketoconazole<br>• Mecamylamine<br>• Methenamine<br>• Milk products<br>• Pancrelipase<br>• Phenytoin<br>• Oral phosphates<br>• Salicylates<br>• Sodium bicarbonate<br>• Sodium fluoride<br>• SPSR<br>• Sucralfate<br>• Tetracyclines<br>• Vitamin D |
| **Dosage** | *Maalox®*<br>• 1 or 2 teaspoons, 4 times a day, taken 20 minutes to 1 hour after meals and at bedtime | *ALternaGEL™*<br>• 1 to 2 teaspoons, as needed, between meals, and at bedtime<br>• May be followed by a sip of water<br><br>*Amphojel®*<br>• 2 teaspoons, followed by a sip of water, 5 to 6 times a day between meals and at bedtime | *Tums E-X®*<br>• 1 or 2 tablets as symptoms occur<br>• Patients should take no more than 10 tablets in a 24-hour period |

# Histamine $H_2$-Receptor Antagonists

| Brand Name | Pepcid® (famotidine) | Zantac® (ranitidine) | Tagamet® (cimetidine) |
|---|---|---|---|
| **Company** | Merck & Co., Inc. | Glaxo Wellcome, Inc. | SmithKline Beecham Pharmaceuticals |
| **Mechanism of Action** | • Inhibit basal and nocturnal gastric secretions by competitively and reversibly inhibiting the action of histamine at the histamine $H_2$-receptors of parietal cells | | |
| **Indications** | • Short-term treatment of active duodenal ulcer<br>• Maintenance treatment of duodenal ulcer at reduced dosage after healing of active ulcer<br>• Short-term treatment of active benign gastric ulcer | | |
| **Contraindication** | • Hypersensitivity to product | | |
| **Adverse Reactions** | • Headache<br>• Dizziness<br>• Constipation<br>• Diarrhea | • *CNS*<br>Headache, and rarely, malaise, dizziness, somnolence, insomnia, vertigo, reversible blurred vision, reversible involuntary motor disturbances<br>• *CV*<br>Arrhythmias<br>• *GI*<br>Constipation, diarrhea, nausea/ vomiting, abdominal pain<br>• *Hepatic*<br>Elevated enzymes<br>• *Integumental*<br>Rash | • *CNS*<br>Headache, dizziness, somnolence, insomnia, vertigo, reversible confused states<br>• *CV*<br>Arrhythmias<br>• *Endocrine*<br>Gynecomastia<br>• *GI*<br>Diarrhea<br>• *Hepatic*<br>Elevated enzymes<br>• *Integumental*<br>Rash<br>• *Renal*<br>Elevated serum creatinine |
| **Drug Interactions** | • None identified | • None identified at recommended doses | • Warfarin<br>• Phenytoin<br>• Propranolol<br>• Nifedipine<br>• Chlordiazepoxide<br>• Diazepam<br>• Certain tricyclic antidepressants<br>• Lidocaine<br>• Theophylline<br>• Metronidazole |

*Continued ...*

# Histamine $H_2$-Receptor Antagonists

| Brand Name | Pepcid® (famotidine) | Zantac® (ranitidine) | Tagamet® (cimetidine) |
|---|---|---|---|
| **Dosage** | *Duodenal—Acute*<br>• 40 mg once a day at bedtime for up to 6 to 8 weeks<br>*Duodenal—Maintenance*<br>• 20 mg once a day at bedtime<br>*Benign Gastric—Acute*<br>• 40 mg once a day at bedtime | *Duodenal—Acute*<br>• 150 mg or 10 mL twice a day<br>—or—<br>300 mg or 20 mL once a day at bedtime<br>*Duodenal—Maintenance*<br>• 150 mg or 10 mL at bedtime<br>*Benign Gastric*<br>• 150 mg or 10 mL twice a day | *Duodenal—Acute*<br>• 800 mg once daily at bedtime for up to 6 to 8 weeks<br>*Duodenal—Maintenance*<br>• 400 mg at bedtime<br>*Benign Gastric*<br>• 800 mg once daily at bedtime for up to 6 weeks |

*Editors' Notes:*

Cimetidine may increase cyclosporine levels and cause nephrotoxicity. Famotidine, ranitidine, and cimetidine are now available over the counter.

# Omeprazole

| | |
|---|---|
| **Brand Name** | Prilosec® |
| **Company** | Astra / Merck Group |
| **Mechanism of Action** | • Suppresses basal and stimulated gastric acid secretion by specific inhibition of the $H^+/K^+$ ATPase enzyme system at the secretory surface of the gastric parietal cell |
| **Indication** | • Short-term treatment of active duodenal ulcer |
| **Contraindication** | • Known hypersensitivity to any component of this agent |
| **Adverse Reactions** | • Headache<br>• Diarrhea<br>• Abdominal pain<br>• Nausea<br>• URI<br>• Dizziness<br>• Vomiting<br>• Rash<br>• Constipation<br>• Cough<br>• Asthenia<br>• Back pain |
| **Drug Interactions** | • Diazepam<br>• Warfarin<br>• Phenytoin<br>• Drugs metabolized via the cytochrome P-450 system (ie, cyclosporine, disulfiram) |
| **Dosage** | • 20 mg once daily for up to 8 weeks |

*Editors' Notes:*

Most effective for established GI disease, but is also the most expensive.

# Sucralfate

| | |
|---|---|
| **Brand Name** | Carafate® |
| **Company** | Marion Merrell Dow Inc. |
| **Mechanism of Action** | • Forms an ulcer-adherent complex that covers the ulcer site and protects it from further attack by acid, pepsin, and bile salts |
| **Indications** | • Short-term treatment of active duodenal ulcers<br>• Maintenance therapy for duodenal ulcers at reduced dosage after healing of acute ulcers |
| **Contraindication** | • None known |
| **Adverse Reactions** | • Constipation<br>• Diarrhea<br>• Nausea/vomiting<br>• Gastric discomfort<br>• Indigestion<br>• Flatulence<br>• Dry mouth<br>• Pruritus<br>• Rash<br>• Dizziness<br>• Sleepiness<br>• Vertigo<br>• Back pain<br>• Headache |
| **Drug Interactions** | • Cimetidine<br>• Phenytoin<br>• Ciprofloxacin<br>• Ranitidine<br>• Digoxin<br>• Tetracycline<br>• Norfloxacin<br>• Theophylline |
| **Dosage** | *Acute Therapy*<br>• 1 g, 4 times a day on an empty stomach for up to 8 weeks |

# Misoprostol

| | |
|---|---|
| **Brand Name** | Cytotec® |
| **Company** | G.D. Searle & Co. |
| **Mechanism of Action** | • Inhibits basal and nocturnal gastric acid secretion by direct action on parietal cells<br>• Enhances natural gastromucosal defense mechanisms and healing by increasing production of gastric mucus and mucosal secretion |
| **Indication** | • Prevention of NSAID-induced gastric ulcers in patients at high risk of complications from gastric ulcer and gastric ulceration |
| **Contraindications** | • Women who are pregnant because misoprostol has abortifacient properties<br>• Should not be used in any woman of child-bearing age unless NSAID therapy is required and patient is at high risk of complications from gastric ulcers. For misoprostol to be prescribed, patient should:<br>  • be capable of complying with effective contraception<br>  • have received oral and written warnings of the hazards of misoprostol<br>  • have had a negative serum pregnancy test within 2 weeks prior to beginning therapy<br>  • begin therapy only on the second or third day of the next normal menstrual period |
| **Adverse Reactions** | • Diarrhea<br>• Abdominal pain<br>• Spotting<br>• Cramps<br>• Hypermenorrhea<br>• Menstrual disorder<br>• Dysmenorrhea<br>• Postmenopausal bleeding<br>• Nausea<br>• Flatulence<br>• Headache<br>• Dyspepsia<br>• Vomiting<br>• Constipation |
| **Drug Interactions** | • None identified |
| **Dosage** | • 200 µg 4 times a day with food for the duration of NSAID therapy |

*Editors' Notes:*

One study suggests that misoprostol may reduce incidence of rejection episodes when combined with cyclosporine and prednisone. Not confirmed in a prospective, randomized trial.

# Chapter 8
# Diuretics

## Diuretics Overview

### Diuretics

- Furosemide
- Bumetanide

# Diuretics Overview

| Agent | Dosage |
|---|---|
| **Furosemide** | *Oral*<br>• Dosage should be individualized<br>• Initial dose is 20 mg to 80 mg given as a single dose<br>• Dose can be raised by 20 mg or 40 mg, given no sooner than 6 to 8 hours after the previous dose, until desired diuretic effect has been achieved<br><br>*Parenteral*<br>• Initial dose is 20 mg to 40 mg given as a single dose, IM or IV. IV injection should be given over 1 to 2 minutes<br>• Dose can be raised by 20 mg, given no sooner than 2 hours after the previous dose, until desired diuretic effect has been achieved<br><br>*Acute Pulmonary Edema*<br>• Initial dose is 40 mg given intravenously over 1 to 2 minutes<br>• Dose can be increased to 80 mg given intravenously if a satisfactory response has not occurred within 1 hour |
| **Bumetanide** | *Oral*<br>• Dosage should be individualized<br>• Initial dosage is 0.5 mg to 2.0 mg given as a single dose on alternate days, or for 3 to 4 days with rest periods of 1 to 2 days<br><br>*Parenteral*<br>• Initial dose is 0.5 mg to 1.0 mg, IM or IV. IV injection should be given over 1 to 2 minutes |

Immuno-suppression
Antimicrobials
Cardiovascular Agents
Antiosteo-porosis Agents
Antiplatelets
Diabetes Agents
Ulcer Treatment
Diuretics
Other Agents

# Diuretics

| Brand Name | Lasix® (furosemide) | Bumex® (bumetanide) |
|---|---|---|
| Company | Hoechst Marion Roussel Pharmaceuticals Inc. | Roche Laboratories |
| Mechanism of Action | • Primarily inhibits the absorption of sodium and chloride in the proximal and distal tubules, as well as in the loop of Henle | • Inhibits sodium reabsorption in the ascending limb of the loop of Henle, as shown by marked water reduction of free-water clearance during hydration and tubular free-water reabsorption during hydropenia |
| Indication | • Edema associated with congestive heart failure, cirrhosis of the liver, and renal disease | |
| Contraindications | • Anuria<br>• Hypersensitivity to agent | • Anuria<br>• Hepatic coma or states of severe electrolyte depletion<br>• Hypersensitivity to agent |
| Adverse Reactions | • *GI*<br>Pancreatitis, jaundice, anorexia, oral and gastric irritation, cramping, diarrhea, constipation, nausea, vomiting<br>• *CNS*<br>Tinnitus and hearing loss, paresthesia, vertigo, dizziness, headache, blurred vision, xanthopsia<br>• *Hematologic*<br>Aplastic anemia, thrombocytopenia, agranulocytosis, hemolytic anemia, leukopenia, anemia<br>• *Dermatologic*<br>Exfoliative dermatis, erythema multiforme, purpura, photosensitivity, urticaria, rash, pruritus<br>• *Other*<br>Orthostatic hypotension, hyperglycemia, glycosuria, hyperuricemia, muscle spasm, weakness, restlessness, urinary bladder spasm, thrombophlebitis, IM injection site pain, fever | • Muscle cramps<br>• Dizziness<br>• Hypotension<br>• Headache<br>• Nausea<br>• Encephalopathy |

*Continued ...*

# Diuretics

| Brand Name | Lasix® (furosemide) | Bumex® (bumetanide) |
|---|---|---|
| **Drug Interactions** | • Aminoglycosides<br>• Ethacrynic acid<br>• Salicylates (high doses)<br>• Succinylcholine<br>• Lithium<br>• Other antihypertensive agents<br>• Norepinephrine<br>• NSAIDs<br>• Indomethacin | • Aminoglycosides<br>• Drugs with nephrotoxic potential<br>• Lithium<br>• Probenecid<br>• Other antihypertensive agents<br>• Indomethacin |
| **Dosage** | *Oral*<br>• Dosage should be individualized<br>• Initial dose is 20 mg to 80 mg given as a single dose<br>• Dose can be raised by 20 mg or 40 mg, given no sooner than 6 to 8 hours after the previous dose, until desired diuretic effect has been achieved<br><br>*Parenteral*<br>• Initial dose is 20 mg to 40 mg given as a single dose, IM or IV. IV injection should be given over 1 to 2 minutes<br>• Dose can be raised by 20 mg, given no sooner than 2 hours after the previous dose, until desired diuretic effect has been achieved<br><br>*Acute Pulmonary Edema*<br>• Initial dose is 40 mg given intravenously over 1 to 2 minutes<br>• Dose can be increased to 80 mg given intravenously if a satisfactory response has not occurred within 1 hour | *Oral*<br>• Dosage should be individualized<br>• Initial dosage is 0.5 mg to 2.0 mg given as a single dose on alternate days or for 3 to 4 days with rest periods of 1 to 2 days<br><br>*Parenteral*<br>• Initial dose is 0.5 mg to 1.0 mg, IM or IV. IV injection should be given over 1 to 2 minutes |

***Editors' Notes:***

Loop diuretics elevate uric acid. Cyclosporine also elevates uric acid, which can lead to gout.

# Chapter 9
# Other Concomitant Agents

## Other Concomitant Agents Overview

## Other Cardiovascular Agents

- Digoxin
- Isosorbide Mononitrate

## Levothyroxine

## Sodium Bicarbonate

## Aquaphor® Ointment

## Octreotide

## Metoclopramide

## Cisapride

## Bethanechol

## Phenytoin

## Warfarin

## Pentoxifylline

## Fludrocortisone

## Potassium

# Other Concomitant Agents Overview

| Agent | Dosage |
|---|---|
| **Other Cardiovascular Agents** | *Digoxin*<br>• Dosage should be individualized according to patient, dosing formulation, and disease state<br>Loading<br>• Peak body digoxin stores of 8 µg/kg to 12 µg/kg should provide therapeutic effect with minimum risk of toxicity for patients with heart failure and normal sinus rhythm<br>• 10 µg/kg to 15 µg/kg may be needed in patients with atrial flutter or fibrillation<br>Maintenance<br>• The following formula can be used to calculate maintenance dose<br>$\text{Loading dose} \times \frac{\text{\% Daily loss}}{100}$<br>% Daily loss = 14 + Ccr/5<br><br>*Isosorbide Mononitrate*<br>• 20 mg (1 tablet), 2 times a day, given 7 hours apart |
| **Levothyroxine** | • Dosage and rate of administration must be individualized<br><br>*Synthroid®*<br>Hypothyroidism<br>• Usual starting dose is 1.6 µg/kg/d, administered once daily<br>• 200 µg/d is usually highest maintenance dose required<br>Myxedema Coma<br>• 300 µg to 500 µg<br>TSH Suppression<br>• Initial dose is followed by daily IV doses of 75 µg to 100 µg until the patient is stable<br><br>*Levothroid®*<br>Hypothyroidism<br>• Usual starting dose is 50 µg/d, with increments of 50 µg/d every 2 to 4 weeks<br>• 100 µg/d to 200 µg/d is usual maintenance range<br>Myxedema Coma<br>• 200 µg to 500 µg given rapidly<br><br>*Levoxine®*<br>Hypothyroidism<br>• Usual starting dose is 25 µg/d to 100 µg/d<br>• A maintenance dose of 100 µg/d to 200 µg/d can be achieved within 2 to 3 weeks<br>Myxedema Coma<br>• Dose may be as little as 12.5 µg/d, with incremental increases of 25 µg/d at 3 to 4 week intervals |
| **Sodium Bicarbonate** | • 1 to 4 tablets QID as needed to replace bicarbonate loss |

*Continued ...*

# Other Concomitant Agents Overview

| Agent | Dosage |
|---|---|
| **Aquaphor® Ointment** | • Applied liberally to affected areas 2 to 3 times a day |
| **Octreotide** | • Initial dosage is 50 μg/d, administered subcutaneously once or twice daily<br>• Number of injections and dosage may be increased gradually based on patient response |
| **Metoclopramide** | *Symptomatic Gastroesophageal Reflux*<br>• 10 mg to 15 mg orally up to QID, 30 minutes before each meal and at bedtime for no longer than 12 weeks<br><br>*Diabetic Gastric Stasis*<br>• 10 mg, 30 minutes before each meal and at bedtime for 2 to 8 weeks<br><br>*Nausea and Vomiting Associated With Cancer Chemotherapy*<br>• 1 mg/kg to 2 mg/kg IV, infused slowly over a period not less than 15 minutes, 30 minutes before beginning chemotherapy and repeated every 2 hours for 2 doses and then every 3 hours for 3 doses<br><br>*Postoperative Nausea and Vomiting*<br>• 10 mg to 20 mg IM, near the end of surgery<br><br>*Facilitate Small Bowel Intubation*<br>• Single 10 mg IV dose administered slowly over a 1- to 2-minute period |
| **Cisapride** | • 10 mg four times daily at least 15 minutes before meals and at bedtime |
| **Bethanechol** | *Oral* (Urecholine®, Duvoid®)<br>• 10 mg to 50 mg, 3 or 4 times a day<br><br>*Subcutaneous (Urecholine)*<br>• 1 mL (5 mg), although some patients respond to as little as 0.5 mL (2.5 mg) initially; minimum effective dose may be repeated 3 or 4 times a day as required |
| **Phenytoin** | *Infatabs®*<br>• 2 Infatabs, 3 times daily, dose then adjusted to suit individual needs<br><br>*Parenteral*<br>• Status epilepticus: Loading IV dose of 10 mg/kg to 15 mg/kg administered slowly, at a rate not exceeding 50 mg/min, followed by a maintenance dose of 100 mg PO or IV every 6 to 8 hours<br>• Neurosurgery: 100 mg to 200 mg IM at approximately 4-hour intervals during surgery and continued postoperatively<br><br>*Suspension*<br>• 1 teaspoon (5 mL), 3 times daily, dose then adjusted to suit individual needs |

*Continued ...*

# Other Concomitant Agents Overview

| Agent | Dosage |
|---|---|
| **Warfarin** | • Dosage must be individualized<br>• Usual initial dosage is 2 mg/d to 5 mg/d, with daily dosage adjustments based on the results of PT determinations<br>• 2 mg/d to 10 mg/d is normal maintenance range |
| **`Pentoxifylline** | • 1 controlled-release tablet (400 mg), 3 times a day with meals, for at least 8 weeks |
| **Fludrocortisone** | *Adrenocortical Insufficiency*<br>• 0.1 mg/d PO<br><br>*Congenital Adrenogenital Syndrome*<br>• 0.1 mg/d PO to 0.2 mg/d PO<br><br>*Idiopathic Orthostatic Hypotension*<br>• 50 μg/d PO to 200 μg/d PO |
| **Potassium** | • Normal adult concentration of serum potassium is 3.5 mmol to 5.0 mmol or mEq per liter, with 4.5 mmol or mEq often used as a reference point<br>• 1 g of potassium acetate provides 10.26 mEq of potassium<br>• 1 g of potassium bicarbonate provides 10 mEq of potassium<br>• 1 g of potassium chloride provides 13.41 mEq of potassium<br>• 1 g of potassium citrate provides 9.26 mEq of potassium<br>• 1 g of potassium gluconate provides 4.27 mEq of potassium |

# Other Cardiovascular Agents

| Brand Name | Lanoxin® (digoxin) | Ismo® (isosorbide mononitrate) |
|---|---|---|
| Company | Glaxo Wellcome Inc. | Wyeth-Ayerst Laboratories |
| Mechanism of Action | • Exerts direct action on cardiac muscle and the specialized conduction system<br>• Also exerts indirect actions on the autonomic nervous system, involving a vagomimetic action and baroreceptor sensitization<br>• Direct and indirect actions result in:<br>  • increase in force and velocity of myocardial systolic contraction<br>  • slowing of heart rate<br>  • decreased conduction velocity through AV node | • Relaxes vascular smooth muscle, with consequent dilatation of peripheral arteries and veins, resulting in peripheral pooling of blood and decreased venous return to the heart<br>• Ultimate effect is a reduction in left ventricular end-diastolic pressure and pulmonary capillary wedge pressure |
| Indications | • Heart failure<br>• Atrial fibrillation<br>• Atrial flutter<br>• Paroxysmal atrial tachycardia | • Prevention of angina pectoris due to coronary artery disease |
| Contraindications | • Ventricular fibrillation<br>• Hypersensitivity to agent | • Allergy to organic nitrates |
| Adverse Reactions | • *Cardiac*<br>Unifocal or multiform ventricular premature contractions, ventricular tachycardia, atrioventricular dissociation, accelerated junctional rhythm, and atrial tachycardia with block<br>• *GI*<br>Anorexia, nausea, vomiting, diarrhea<br>• *CNS*<br>Visual disturbances, headache, weakness, dizziness, apathy, psychosis<br>• *Other*<br>Gynecomastia | • Headache<br>• Dizziness<br>• Nausea, vomiting |

*Continued ...*

# Other Cardiovascular Agents

| Brand Name | Lanoxin® (digoxin) | Ismo® (isosorbide mononitrate) |
|---|---|---|
| **Drug Interactions** | • Potassium-depleting corticosteroids and diuretics<br>• Calcium<br>• Quinidine<br>• Verapamil<br>• Amiodarone<br>• Propafenone<br>• Certain antibiotics<br>• Propantheline<br>• Diphenoxylate<br>• Antacids<br>• Kaolin-pectin<br>• Sulfasalazine<br>• Neomycin<br>• Cholestyramine<br>• Certain anticancer agents<br>• Thyroid<br>• Sympathomimetics<br>• Succinylcholine<br>• Beta-blockers/calcium channel blockers | • Other vasodilators, especially alcohol<br>• Calcium channel blockers |
| **Dosage** | • Dosage should be individualized according to patient, dosing formulation, and disease state<br><br>*Loading Dose*<br>• Peak body digoxin stores of 8 µg/kg to 12 µg/kg should provide therapeutic effect with minimum risk of toxicity for patients with heart failure and normal sinus rhythm<br>• 10 µg/kg to 15 µg/kg may be needed in patients with atrial flutter or fibrillation<br><br>*Maintenance Dose*<br>• The following formula can be used to calculate maintenance dose<br>$\text{Loading dose} \times \frac{\%\ \text{Daily loss}}{100}$<br>% Daily loss = 14 + Ccr/5 | • 20 mg (1 tablet), 2 times a day, given 7 hours apart |

# Levothyroxine

| Brand Name | Synthroid® | Levothroid® | Levoxine® |
|---|---|---|---|
| Company | Knoll Laboratories | Forest Laboratories, Inc. | Daniels Pharmaceuticals, Inc. |
| Mechanism of Action | • Provide thyroid hormone that is structurally and functionally equivalent to an endogenously produced thyroid hormone | | |
| Indications | • Replacement or supplemental therapy for patients with hypothyroidism<br>• Pituitary TSH suppressant<br>• Diagnostic agent in suppression tests | | • Replacement or supplemental therapy for patients with hypothyroidism |
| Contraindications | • Diagnosed, but uncorrected adrenal cortical insufficiency<br>• Untreated thyrotoxicosis<br>• Hypersensitivity to any component of drug<br>• Myocardial infarction | | |
| Adverse Reactions | • Adverse reactions other than those indicative of hyperthyroidism due to overdosage are rare<br>• Signs and symptoms of hyperthyroidism include:<br>Weight loss, palpitation, nervousness, diarrhea or abdominal cramps, sweating, tachycardia, cardiac arrhythmias, angina pectoris, tremors, headache, insomnia, intolerance to heat, and fever | | |
| Drug Interactions | • Oral anticoagulants<br>• Insulin or oral hypoglycemics<br>• Cholestyramine<br>• Estrogen, oral contraceptives | | |
| Dosage | • Dosage and rate of administration must be individualized according to patient response<br><br>*Hypothyroidism*<br>• Usual starting dose is 1.6 µg/kg/d administered once daily<br>• 200 µg/d is usually highest maintenance dose required<br><br>*Myxedema Coma*<br>• 300 µg to 500 µg<br>• Initial dose is followed by daily IV doses of 75 µg to 100 µg until patient is stable<br><br>*TSH Suppression*<br>• Doses > 2 µg/kg/d are usually required | • Dosage and rate of administration must be individualized according to patient response<br><br>*Hypothyroidism*<br>• Usual starting dose is 50 µg/d, with increments of 50 µg/d every 2 to 4 weeks<br>• 100 µg/d to 200 µg/d is usual maintenance range<br><br>*Myxedema Coma*<br>• 200 µg to 500 µg given rapidly | • Dosage and rate of administration must be individualized according to patient response<br><br>*Hypothyroidism*<br>• Usual starting dose is 25 µg/d to 100 µg/d<br>• A maintenance dose of 100 µg/d to 200 µg/d can be achieved within 2 to 3 weeks<br><br>*Myxedema Coma*<br>• Dose may be as little as 12.5 µg/d, with incremental increases of 25 µg/d at 3 to 4 week intervals |

# Sodium Bicarbonate

| | |
|---|---|
| **Mechanism of Action** | • Replaces bicarbonate in bladder-drained pancreas |
| **Indication** | • Relief of acid indigestion, sour stomach, or heartburn |
| **Dosage** | • 1 to 4 tablets QID as needed to replace bicarbonate loss |

*Editors' Notes:*

After pancreas transplantation, up to 10 to 12 tablets per day are necessary to prevent metabolic acidosis. Monitor $CO_2$ levels.

Immuno-suppression | Antimicrobials | Cardiovascular Agents | Antiosteo-porosis Agents | Antiplatelets | Diabetes Agents | Ulcer Treatment | Diuretics | Other Agents

# Aquaphor® Ointment

| | |
|---|---|
| **Brand Name** | • Aquaphor® Ointment<br>• Aquaphor® Antibiotic Formula<br>• Aquaphor® Natural Healing Ointment |
| **Company** | Beiersdorf Inc. |
| **Mechanism of Action** | • Absorbs several times its own weight, forming smooth, creamy, water-in-oil emulsions |
| **Indications** | • Accelerated healing of severely dry skin, cracked skin, and minor burns<br>• To reduce skin wound healing time and risk of infection<br>• Follow-up skin treatment for patients undergoing radiation therapy or other drying/burning medical therapies |
| **Precautions** | • For external use only<br>• Avoid contact with eyes<br>• Should not be applied over third-degree burns, deep or puncture wounds, infections, or lacerations |
| **Dosage** | • Applied liberally to affected areas 2 to 3 times a day |

*Editors' Notes:*

Very useful in diabetic patients.

# Octreotide

| | |
|---|---|
| **Brand Name** | Sandostatin® |
| **Company** | Novartis |
| **Mechanism of Action** | • Exerts pharmacological actions similar to the hormone somatostatin including:<br>•suppression of serotonin and gastroenteropancreatic peptides (gastrin, vasoactive intestinal peptide, insulin, glucagon, secretin, motilin, and pancreatic polypeptide)<br>•suppression of growth hormone<br>•suppression of the LH response to GnRH |
| **Indication** | • Control of symptoms in patients with metastatic carcinoid (severe diarrhea and flushing episodes) and vasoactive intestinal peptide-secreting tumors (profuse watery diarrhea) |
| **Contraindication** | • Known hypersensitivity to any component of this agent |
| **Adverse Reactions** | • Gallstones or sludge<br>• Nausea<br>• Injection site pain<br>• Diarrhea<br>• Abdominal pain/discomfort<br>• Loose stools<br>• Vomiting |
| **Drug Interactions** | • Therapy used to control glycemic states (sulfonylureas, insulin, diazoxide, beta-blockers)<br>• Agents used to control electrolyte balance<br>• Octreotide has been associated with alterations in nutrient absorption, and thus may have an effect on any orally administered drug |
| **Dosage** | • Initial dosage is 50 µg/d, administered subcutaneously once or twice daily<br>• Number of injections and dosage may be increased gradually based on patient response |

*Editors' Notes:*

Prospective, randomized trial did not show a benefit after pancreas transplantation. Octreotide lowers cyclosporine-A levels and may cause escape rejection if cyclosporine levels are not carefully monitored.

# Metoclopramide

| | |
|---|---|
| **Brand Name** | Reglan® |
| **Company** | Roberts Pharmaceutical Corp. |
| **Mechanism of Action** | • Increases tone and amplitude of gastric contractions, relaxes the pyloric sphincter and the duodenal bulb, and increases peristalsis of the duodenum and jejunum, possibly by sensitizing tissues to the action of acetylcholine, resulting in accelerated gastric emptying and intestinal transit |
| **Indications** | • Short-term treatment of symptomatic gastroesophageal reflux<br>• Relief of symptoms associated with acute and recurrent diabetic gastric stasis<br>• Prophylaxis of nausea and vomiting associated with cancer chemotherapy<br>• Prophylaxis of postoperative nausea and vomiting<br>• To facilitate small bowel intubation<br>• To stimulate gastric emptying and intestinal transit of barium during radiologic examination |
| **Contraindications** | • Conditions in which stimulation of gastrointestinal motility might be dangerous (e.g., presence of gastrointestinal hemorrhage, mechanical obstruction, or perforation)<br>• Pheochromocytoma<br>• Epilepsy<br>• Hypersensitivity to any component of this agent |
| **Adverse Reactions** | • *CNS*<br>Restlessness, drowsiness, fatigue, lassitude, insomnia, headache, confusion, dizziness, mental depression<br>• *Extrapyramidal Reactions*<br>Acute dystonic reactions, Parkinsonian-like symptoms<br>• *Endocrine Disturbances*<br>Galactorrhea, amenorrhea, gynecomastia, impotence secondary to hyperprolactinemia, fluid retention secondary to transient elevation of aldosterone<br>• *Cardiovascular*<br>Hypotension, hypertension, supraventricular tachycardia and bradycardia<br>• *Gastrointestinal*<br>Nausea and bowel disturbances, primarily diarrhea<br>• *Hepatic*<br>Rarely, cases of hepatotoxicity<br>• *Renal*<br>Urinary frequency and incontinence<br>• *Hematologic*<br>Few cases of neutropenia, leukopenia, or agranulocytosis<br>• *Allergic Reactions*<br>Few cases of rash, urticaria, or bronchospasm |

*Continued ...*

# Metoclopramide

| | |
|---|---|
| **Drug Interactions** | • Anticholinergic drugs<br>• Narcotic analgesics<br>• Alcohol, sedatives, hypnotics, narcotics, tranquilizer<br>• MAO inhibitors<br>• Digoxin<br>• Acetaminophen<br>• Tetracycline<br>• Levodopa<br>• Ethanol<br>• Insulin |
| **Dosage** | *Symptomatic Gastroesophageal Reflux*<br>• 10 mg to 15 mg orally up to QID, 30 minutes before each meal and at bedtime for no longer than 12 weeks<br><br>*Diabetic Gastric Stasis*<br>• 10 mg, 30 minutes before each meal and at bedtime for 2 to 8 weeks<br><br>*Nausea and Vomiting Associated with Cancer Chemotherapy*<br>• 1 mg/kg to 2 mg/kg IV, infused slowly over a period not less than 15 minutes, 30 minutes before beginning chemotherapy and repeated every 2 hours for 2 doses and then every 3 hours for 3 doses<br><br>*Postoperative Nausea and Vomiting*<br>• 10 mg to 20 mg IM, near the end of surgery<br><br>*Facilitate Small Bowel Intubation*<br>• Single 10 mg IV dose administered slowly over a 1- to 2-minute period |

*Editors' Notes:*

Extrapyramidal side effects make this drug less useful than cisapride. Neurologic toxicity is extremely common posttransplant.

# Cisapride

| | |
|---|---|
| **Brand Name** | Propulsid® |
| **Company** | Janssen Pharmaceutica |
| **Mechanism of Action** | • Enhances release of acetylcholine at the myenteric plexus, resulting in gastrointestinal motility |
| **Indication** | • Symptomatic treatment of nocturnal heartburn due to gastroesophageal reflux |
| **Contraindications** | • Concomitant use of ketoconazole, itraconazole, miconazole, or troleandomycin<br>• Conditions in which stimulation of gastrointestinal motility might be dangerous (e.g., presence of gastrointestinal hemorrhage, mechanical obstruction, or perforation)<br>• Hypersensitivity to any component of this agent |
| **Adverse Reactions** | • Dizziness<br>• Vomiting<br>• Pharyngitis<br>• Chest pain<br>• Fatigue<br>• Back pain<br>• Depression<br>• Dehydration<br>• Myalgia |
| **Drug Interactions** | • Ketoconazole<br>• Itraconazole<br>• Miconazole<br>• Troleandomycin<br>• Anticholinergic compounds<br>• Cimetidine |
| **Dosage** | • 10 mg four times daily at least 15 minutes before meals and at bedtime |

# Bethanechol

| Brand Name | Urecholine® | Duvoid® |
|---|---|---|
| Company | Merck & Co., Inc. | Roberts Pharmaceutical Corp. |
| Mechanism of Action | • Produces the effects of a stimulated parasympathetic nervous system, increasing the tone of the detrusor urinae muscle leading to the production of a contraction strong enough to initiate micturition and empty the bladder | |
| Indication | • Treatment of acute postoperative and postpartum nonobstructive (functional) urinary retention and for neurogenic atony of the urinary bladder with retention | |
| Contraindications | • Hypersensitivity to any components of this agent<br>• Hyperthyroidism<br>• Peptic ulcer<br>• Latent or active bronchial asthma<br>• Pronounced bradycardia or hypotension<br>• Vasomotor instability<br>• Coronary artery disease<br>• Epilepsy<br>• Parkinsonism | |
| Adverse Reactions | • *Body as Whole*<br>Malaise<br>• *Digestive*<br>Abdominal cramps or discomfort, colicky pain, nausea and belching, diarrhea, borborygmi, salivation<br>• *Renal*<br>Urinary urgency<br>• *CNS*<br>Headache<br>• *Cardiovascular*<br>Fall in blood pressure with reflex tachycardia, vasomotor response<br>• *Skin*<br>Flushing producing a feeling of warmth, sensation of heat around the face, sweating<br>• *Respiratory*<br>Bronchial constriction, asthmatic attacks<br>• *Other*<br>Lacrimation, miosis | |
| Drug Interaction | • Ganglion blocking compounds | |
| Dosage | *Oral*<br>• 10 mg to 50 mg, 3 or 4 times a day<br><br>*Subcutaneous (Urecholine)*<br>• 1 mL (5 mg), although some patients respond to as little as 0.5 mL (2.5 mg) initially; minimum effective dose may be repeated 3 or 4 times a day as required | |

***Editors' Notes:***

Useful for some diabetic patients with neurogenic bladder dysfunction.

# Phenytoin

| | |
|---|---|
| **Brand Name** | Dilantin® |
| **Company** | Parke-Davis |
| **Mechanism of Action** | • Stabilizes the threshold against hyperexcitability caused by excessive stimulation or environmental changes capable of reducing membrane sodium gradient, possibly by promoting sodium efflux from neurons |
| **Indications** | • Control of generalized tonic-clonic (grand mal) and complex partial (psychomotor, temporal lobe) seizures<br>• Prevention of seizures during or following neurosurgery<br>*Parenteral*<br>• Status epilepticus of the grand mal type |
| **Contraindication** | • Hypersensitivity to phenytoin or other hydantoins |
| **Adverse Reactions** | • Nystagmus<br>• Ataxia<br>• Slurred speech<br>• Decreased coordination and mental confusion<br>• Dizziness<br>• Insomnia<br>• Transient nervousness<br>• Motor twitchings<br>• Headache |
| **Drug Interactions** | • *Increase Phenytoin Serum Levels*<br>Acute alcohol intake, amiodarone, chloramphenicol, chlordiazepoxide, diazepam, dicumarol, disulfiram, estrogens, $H_2$-antagonists, halothane, isoniazid, methylphenidate, phenothiazines, phenylbutazone, salicylates, succinimides, sulfonamides, tolbutamide, trazodone<br>• *Decrease Phenytoin Serum Levels*<br>Carbamazepine, chronic alcohol abuse, reserpine, sucralfate, molindon hydrochloride, antacids containing calcium<br>• *May Increase or Decrease Phenytoin Serum Levels*<br>Phenobarbital, sodium valproate, valproic acid<br>• *Others*<br>Tricyclic antidepressants, corticosteroids, coumarin anticoagulants, digitoxin, doxycycline, furosemide, oral contraceptives, quinidine, rifampin, theophylline, vitamin D |
| **Dosage** | *Infatabs®*<br>• 2 Infatabs, 3 times daily, dose then adjusted to suit individual needs<br><br>*Parenteral*<br>• Status epilepticus: Loading IV dose of 10 mg/kg to 15 mg/kg administered slowly, at a rate not exceeding 50 mg/min, followed by a maintenance dose of 100 mg PO or IV every 6 to 8 hours<br>• Neurosurgery: 100 mg to 200 mg IM at approximately 4-hour intervals during surgery and continued postoperatively<br><br>*Suspension*<br>• 1 teaspoon (5 mL), 3 times daily, dose then adjusted to suit individual needs |

# Warfarin

| | |
|---|---|
| **Brand Name** | Coumadin® |
| **Company** | DuPont Pharma |
| **Mechanism of Action** | • Inhibits the synthesis of vitamin K-dependent coagulation factors, leading to sequential depression of Factors VII, IX, X, and II |
| **Indications** | • Prophylaxis and/or treatment of venous thrombosis and its extension, pulmonary embolism, and atrial fibrillation with embolization<br>• Adjunct in the prophylaxis of systemic embolism after myocardial infarction |
| **Contraindications** | • Pregnancy<br>• Hemorrhagic tendencies or blood dyscrasias<br>• Recent or contemplated surgery<br>• Bleeding tendencies associated with active ulceration or overt bleeding<br>• Threatened abortion<br>• Inadequate laboratory facilities<br>• Spinal puncture<br>• Major regional, lumbar block anesthesia<br>• Malignant hypertension |
| **Adverse Reactions** | • Hemorrhage from any tissue or organ<br>• Necrosis of skin and other tissues<br>• Alopecia<br>• Urticaria<br>• Dermatitis<br>• Fever<br>• Nausea<br>• Diarrhea<br>• Abdominal cramping<br>• Cramping<br>• Systemic cholesterol microembolization<br>• "Purple toes" syndrome<br>• Cholestatic hepatic injury<br>• Hypersensitivity reactions |
| **Drug Interactions** | *Increase PT Time*<br>• Alcohol<br>• Allopurinol<br>• Aminosalicylic acid<br>• Amiodarone HCl<br>• Anabolic steroids<br>• Anesthetics, inhal.<br>• Antibiotics<br>• Bromelains<br>• Chenodiol<br>• Chloral hydrate<br>• Chlorpropamide<br>• Chymotrypsin<br>• Cimetidine<br>• Clofibrate<br>• Dextran<br>• Dextrothyroxine<br>• Diazoxide<br>• Diflunisal<br>• Diuretics<br>• Disulfiram<br>• Ethacrynic acid<br>• Fenoprofen<br>• Glucagon<br>• Hepatotoxic drugs<br>• Ibuprofen<br>• Indomethacin<br>• Influenza vaccine<br>• Lovastatin<br>• Mefenamic acid<br>• Methyldopa<br>• Methylphenidate<br>• Metronidazole<br>• Miconazole<br>• MAO inhibitors<br>• Nalidixic acid<br>• Naproxen<br>• Narcotics, prolonged<br>• Pentoxifylline<br>• Phenylbutazone<br>• Phenytoin<br>• Propafenone<br>• Pyrazolones<br>• Quinidine<br>• Quinine<br>• Quinolones<br>• Ranitidine<br>• Salicylates<br>• Sulfinpyrazone<br>• Sulfonamides<br>• Sulindac<br>• Tamoxifen<br>• Thyroid drugs<br>• Tolbutamide<br>• TMP/SMX |

*Continued ...*

# Warfarin

| | |
|---|---|
| **Drug Interactions** (Continued) | *Decrease PT Time*<br>• Adrenocortical steroids<br>• Alcohol<br>• Aminoglutethimide<br>• Antacids<br>• Antihistamines<br>• Barbiturates<br>• Carbamazepine<br>• Chloral hydrate<br>• Chlordiazepoxide<br>• Cholestyramine<br>• Diuretics<br>• Diets high in vitamin K<br>• Ethchlorvynol<br>• Glutethimide<br>• Griseofluvin<br>• Haloperidol<br>• Meprobamate<br>• Nafcillin<br>• Oral contraceptives<br>• Paraldehyde<br>• Primidone<br>• Ranitidine<br>• Rifampin<br>• Sucralfate<br>• Trazodone<br>• Vitamin C |
| **Dosage** | • Dosage must be individualized<br>• Usual initial dosage is 2 mg/d to 5 mg/d, with daily dosage adjustments based on the results of PT determinations<br>• 2 mg/d to 10 mg/d is normal maintenance range |

# Pentoxifylline

| | |
|---|---|
| **Brand Name** | Trental® |
| **Company** | Hoechst Marion Roussel Pharmaceuticals Inc. |
| **Mechanism of Action** | • Improves flow properties of blood by decreasing its viscosity |
| **Indication** | • Treatment of patients with intermittent claudication on the basis of chronic occlusive arterial disease |
| **Contraindications** | • Known hypersensitivity to any component of this agent or methylxanthines (caffeine, theophylline, theobromine) |
| **Adverse Reactions** | • *Cardiovascular*<br>Angina/chest pain, arrhythmias/palpitation, flushing<br>• *Digestive*<br>Abdominal discomfort, belching/flatus/bloating, diarrhea, dyspepsia, nausea, vomiting<br>• *CNS*<br>Agitation/nervousness, dizziness, drowsiness, headache, insomnia, tremor, blurred vision |
| **Drug Interactions** | • Anticoagulants or platelet aggregation inhibitors<br>• Antihypertensives (because small decreases in blood pressure may occur during treatment with pentoxifylline) |
| **Dosage** | • 1 controlled-release tablet (400 mg), 3 times a day with meals, for at least 8 weeks |

# Fludrocortisone

| | |
|---|---|
| **Brand Name** | Florinef® |
| **Company** | Apothecon |
| **Mechanism of Action** | • Acts on the distal tubules to increase potassium excretion, hydrogen ion excretion, and sodium reabsorption and subsequent water retention |
| **Indications** | • Treatment of adrenocortical insufficiency, chronic primary and chronic secondary<br>• Treatment of congenital adrenogenital syndrome<br>• Treatment of idiopathic orthostatic hypotension<br>• Treatment and diagnosis of acidosis in renal tubular disorders |
| **Contraindications/ Medical Problems** | • Known hypersensitivity to any component of this agent<br>• Cardiac disease<br>• Congestive heart failure<br>• Peripheral edema<br>• Renal function impairment, except in treatment of renal tubular acidosis<br>• Acute glomerulonephritis<br>• Hepatic function impairment<br>• Hypothyroidism or hyperthyroidism<br>• Chronic nephritis<br>• Osteoporosis |
| **Adverse Reactions** | • Generalized anaphylaxis<br>• Congestive heart failure<br>• Dizziness<br>• Headache<br>• Severe or continuing hypokalemic syndrome |
| **Drug Interactions** | • Digitalis glycosides<br>• Hepatic enzyme inducers<br>• Hypokalemia-causing medications<br>• Lithium<br>• Sodium-containing medications or foods |
| **Dosage** | *Adrenocortical Insufficiency*<br>• 0.1 mg/d PO<br><br>*Congenital Adrenogenital Syndrome*<br>• 0.1 mg/d PO to 0.2 mg/d PO<br><br>*Idiopathic Orthostatic Hypotension*<br>• 50 µg/d PO to 200 µg/d PO |

*Editors' Notes:*

Useful for treating hyperkalemia due to tacrolimus and cyclosporine. Also useful for orthostatic hypotension in diabetic autonomic neuropathy.

# Potassium

| | |
|---|---|
| **Brand Name** | Various |
| **Mechanism of Action** | • Potassium is the predominant cation within cells and, as such, high intracellular potassium concentrations are necessary for numerous cellular metabolic processes |
| **Indication** | • Treatment and prophylaxis of hypokalemia |
| **Contraindications** | • Known hypersensitivity to potassium<br>• Hyperkalemia |
| **Adverse Reactions** | • Hyperkalemia<br>• Contact irritation of the alimentary tract<br>• Diarrhea<br>• Nausea<br>• Stomach pain, discomfort, or gas<br>• Vomiting |
| **Drug Interactions** | • Amphotericin B<br>• Corticosteroids<br>• Corticotropin<br>• Gentamicin<br>• Penicillins<br>• Polymyxin B<br>• ACE inhibitors<br>• NSAIDs<br>• Beta-blockers<br>• Blood from blood bank<br>• Cyclosporine<br>• Potassium-sparing diuretics<br>• Heparin<br>• Low-salt milk<br>• Potassium-containing medications<br>• Salt substitutes<br>• Anticholinergics<br>• Calcium salts<br>• Digitalis glycosides in presence of heart block<br>• Thiazide diuretics<br>• Exchange resins, sodium cycle<br>• Insulin<br>• Sodium bicarbonate<br>• Laxatives |
| **Dosage** | • Normal adult concentration of serum potassium is 3.5 mmol to 5.0 mmol or mEq per liter, with 4.5 mmol or mEq often used as a reference point<br>• 1 g of potassium acetate provides 10.26 mEq of potassium<br>• 1 g of potassium bicarbonate provides 10 mEq of potassium<br>• 1 g of potassium chloride provides 13.41 mEq of potassium<br>• 1 g of potassium citrate provides 9.26 mEq of potassium<br>• 1 g of potassium gluconate provides 4.27 mEq of potassium |

# Index